Nursing Management for Patient Care

Nursing Management for Patient Care

Second Edition

Marjorie Beyers, R.N., Ph.D.

Director, Evanston Hospital School of Nursing
Evanston, Illinois

Carole Phillips, R.N., M.S.

Formerly Instructor, Evanston Hospital School of Nursing
Evanston, Illinois

Little, Brown and Company   Boston

Preface

The nursing profession has become complex and differentiated in the numerous types of specialties and levels of practice it encompasses. Nurses are becoming increasingly important in the health-care industry and can be found in various positions in every type of health-care agency. For the most part, nurses are employed by health-care agencies and consequently provide their services within the context of an organization. That organizational identity as well as the differentiation among the levels of nurses employed by a given health-care agency requires that nurses become managers. The differences in levels of nursing knowledge and practice are concomitant with the different levels of management roles that nurses fulfill. Some nurses manage patient care for a discrete number of patients, others manage both nurses and patient care, and yet others manage entire nursing or nursing-related departments in agencies within the health-care industry.

This book has been written expressly for the nurse who is making the transition from learning about individualized patient care to becoming a manager of that care within an organization. The newly graduated nurse often perceives a dichotomy between the role behaviors expected of a student and those expected of an employee in a health-care agency. The differences perceived are related to the emphasis on patient care. In most basic nursing education programs emphasis is placed on the nurse-patient relationship and related behaviors of the nurse in giving individualized patient care. As an employee, the nurse finds that the emphasis shifts to include managing other levels of nursing personnel and working with medical personnel in an organizational structure. The nurse who is beginning a first position in nursing must continue to develop role behaviors related to giving individualized patient care while also adjusting to the new role behaviors of a manager, which may or may not have been included in the basic nursing education program. It is our belief that the nurse who adjusts successfully to becoming a manager can better apply the knowledge and expertise in giving patient care that are gained in the basic nursing program.

This book has been developed on the premise that student nurses learn a great deal about human behavior in a basic nursing education program and that such knowledge can be used as the foundation for learning management theories and principles. The beginning student of management can extend the knowledge of human behavior from the dimension of the nurse-patient relationship along a continuum that eventually can incorporate managing a large component of a health-care agency. Nurses can apply their knowledge and understanding of human behaviors in the nurse-patient relationship to the behaviors of people in organizations. Just as a person has a distinct personality, an organization also has a distinct personality that can be studied through the aegis of management.

The study of management in basic nursing education programs often focuses on leadership rather than on generalized management theories. We believe that nurses must be both leaders and managers and that knowledge of management theories and principles is necessary in order to give nursing care effectively within a health-care agency. Nurses who work in organizations should know how those organizations are structured, how they function, and how one can use the components of an organization to support active involvement in the dynamic processes of giving nursing care.

Management theories are important not only for maintaining effective nursing care but also for developing improvements in the nursing-care delivery system. Nursing care takes place within the health-care delivery system, and the total health-care industry is changing rapidly. As part of this rapidly changing industry, nurses should assume a prominent role in continually improving not only nursing care but also the health-care delivery system.

The basic premise of this book is that all nurses are managers. The text has been written as an introduction to management for use by those who are studying management theories and principles in basic nursing education programs and as a reference for the nurse who is learning to become a manager in the work situation. The theories and principles of management discussed provide a basis for understanding how organizations are structured and how people behave in organizations. The content of the book will enable the reader to study and analyze nursing management practices. In addition, the theories presented can be used as tools for working with others in the management of nursing care in a health-care agency. When working in an organization the nurse must learn to give expert, individualized patient care within the context of the organization and to use management theories in order to be effective within the organization.

Nursing Management for Patient Care is divided into three parts. Part I deals with general management theories on organizations and organizational practices. Content in the first part is designed to provide the reader with a frame of reference about organizations that gives substance to the content presented in the second part. More specific information about management techniques in use on a day-to-day basis is included in Part II. Behaviors of managers who are functioning in patient-care units in hospitals are emphasized here, although the content is not exclusive to hospital management. Each chapter in the first and second parts of the book can be studied independently of the other chapters. Part III includes case studies designed to help the reader develop skills in solving management problems. That part gives the reader an opportunity to synthesize the content included in the first two parts by analyzing problems commonly found in nursing management. The cases provide a practical vehicle for the study of management as applied to the work situation.

The health-care industry is a complex business comprising many different types of health-care agencies. Some of those agencies are representative of new developments in the health-care delivery system and others are an admixture of traditional and progressive organizations. Most hospitals, for example, use a variety of traditional and progressive organizational strategies that are appropriate for a given setting. All the different agencies within the health-care industry require managers who deal with the problems that exist in every organization. Some problems are related to how people work together, others to the specific needs of an organization, and yet others to change processes ongoing in the health-care industry. The nurse-manager must have a flexible mind to analyze and solve those problems successfully. This book should serve to broaden the nurse's perspective of management and organizations and should increase the reader's ability to identify and resolve management problems.

We are grateful to the many people who assisted in the revision of this manuscript, particularly June Werner whose advice was invaluable, Barbara Blatecky who provided library resources, and all the persons mentioned in the previous edition who contributed to the initial writing. Many of the fine illustrations by Lou Pearson have been retained in this edition. We also express appreciation to the students who gave us helpful and challenging reviews of the manuscript and to our families who provided support and encouragement during the progress of this work.

M. B.
C. P.

Contents

I. A Framework
of Management

1. Health-Care Organizations

You have selected a career in nursing. This career places you in the mainstream of the health-care industry, which exists for the purpose of providing services to individuals. As a nurse, you are primarily concerned with giving care based on your nursing knowledge and expertise. In becoming a nurse, you have learned how a person functions, psychologically and physiologically, and you have learned about the types of problems a person may encounter throughout the life cycle. You have learned that the essence of nursing care is helping people achieve or maintain a maximum state of "wellness" or health. In studying the process of nursing care, you have learned concepts and methods that can be applied in patient-care situations to help individuals achieve a maximum state of health. In order to achieve your maximum potential as a professional nurse, you must function within a health-care system that shares your goals in giving patient care. Functioning within this health-care system places you in an organization that supports you and that provides you with the environment and resources you need to administer nursing care.

While the functions of nursing care are carried out within the context of the nurse-patient relationship, the environment in which this takes place greatly influences the nature of that relationship. The environment in which you give patient care is usually a health-service agency, such as a hospital, a clinic, or some other type of organization that exists to provide care for patients. When working within such organizations, you rely on and cooperate with other health professionals. You also work with people who provide the supporting services that the care-givers require to carry out their specialized functions. In so doing, you share a common goal with others who have different academic preparation and specialized expertise; these others include physicians, physical therapists, occupational therapists, speech therapists, administrators, accountants, systems analysts, and housekeeping specialists, to name a few. You may relate directly to some of these persons, or you may use the services they provide without having direct personal contact with them. As a nurse, your primary function remains that of giving patient care, and you tend to know about the functions of other professionals through your day-by-day interactions with them in the patient-care setting. You relate only indirectly to those who work "behind the scenes," even though the environment in which you work is influenced by their functions.

Most nurses are employed by health-care agencies, and when a nurse accepts employment in a health-care agency, that nurse becomes a member of an organization. The organization employs the nurse because it requires the services that the nurse can provide for patients. The nurse seeks employment in the organization because that organization provides the medium in which nursing care can be given. Thus, there is an interdependence between the nurse and the employing organization. In order to implement the work necessary for patient care, the organization generally employs a number of other types of health professionals with different kinds of patient-care expertise. Each of these professionals also requires the supporting services of the organization to administer specialized care. In this respect, the organization provides for the interaction of a number of different professionals who cooperate in giving care and who are dependent on one another to provide the full spectrum of services that any given patient requires. There is, then, a mutual interdependence of all of the members of the organization on each other and on the organization. The professionals have expectations of the organization and of each other in this mutual relationship. Likewise, the organization has expectations of all of its members.

People employed by organizations expect the organization to provide a safe, efficient workplace and the mechanisms necessary to perform specialized functions. They also expect that the employing organization will provide them with a sense of identity and with the necessities of livelihood, such as salary and fringe benefits. The institution provides this medium for practice and expects that its members will contribute to the growth and maintenance of the organization in a complementary and productive manner. The organization, for example, expects that employed nurses will be competent in giving patient care and that they will use the health-care agency's material and human resources effectively and efficiently in administering this care. As members of organizations, nurses should know how organizations are formed, how they are maintained, and how people work together within them.

Organizations

Organizations are formed to meet the needs of society. Some organizations provide public services required by society. Others provide people with goods and products, such as automobiles and clothing. All organizations have certain things in common. To survive, they must have a purpose and well-defined objectives, and they must produce something that is useful to society. To produce, organizations require a number of resources, including manpower, physical resources such as buildings and equipment, expendable resources such as materials and supplies, and capital. All organizations have some form of structure that designates how employees work together. The structure or design influences the way that people behave in managing the use of resources to achieve organizational purposes.

There are many different types of organizations, and these differ in purpose and in the amount or kind of resources needed to achieve this purpose. Organizations that use tools and machines predominantly in pursuing their objectives are technologically oriented. Those that use people as their predominant resource are called labor-intensive. Examples of labor-intensive organizations are schools and hospitals. Both schools and hospitals are public-service organizations that exist to meet a public need; schools meet the need for education, and hospitals meet the need for health care. Another difference in types of organizations is whether they are intended to produce a profit. An organization that produces automobiles intends to produce a profit. Public-service institutions, such as schools and hospitals, are usually nonprofit organizations.

A given organization, although it may be independent, can be part of a larger industry. An automobile plant, for example, is part of the larger auto industry. Hospitals are part of the health-care industry. Organizations are affected by other components of their industry in many ways. They may be in competition with one another for acquiring both resources and customers. These organizations can be publicly or privately owned and can vary in size, strength, structure, philosophy, and specific goals. New developments in one organization may affect other organizations in the industry and external factors such as state or federal legislation may affect all of the organizations within the industry. In such matters as state and federal legislation, the public tends to think of the industry as a whole because it is the industry, rather than a particular agency, that meets the needs of the public.

Use of the term *health-care industry* is of recent origin. There are many types of health-care agencies and organizations within this industry. Traditionally health-care agencies have been classified as either official agencies or voluntary agencies. The official or public agencies are tax-supported, and the voluntary agencies are supported primarily by private funds. Most voluntary agencies are nonprofit and tax-free organizations, but there are private health-care agencies that are profit-making. Examples of public or official agencies are the Public Health Service hospitals, the Veterans Administration hospital system, the armed forces hospitals, and the Indian Health Service. The community hospital is the most commonly found example of the voluntary, nonprofit health-care agency. In general, the hospital is the central core of the health-care service industry, but new types of health-care agencies are emerging.

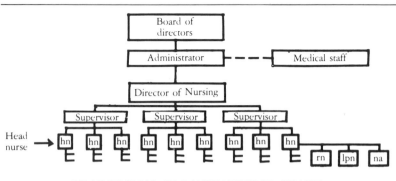

TRADITIONAL ORGANIZATIONAL CHART

The particular purposes of an organization stem from the reasons why the organization was originally founded and evolve from that point according to the needs of the community served by the organization. Community hospitals, for example, usually have originated from a realization of need by citizens in the community. In many instances, the citizens participated in planning, in raising funds, or in developing projects that led to the founding of the hospital. The authority for founding the hospital organization is granted by the state in the form of a charter. This charter includes a statement of the purposes and functions of the hospital, which must be fulfilled in the public interest through the administration of the hospital.

Public involvement in a community hospital continues after the hospital is established. The hospital's board of directors or trustees is usually made up of community members who are responsible for the administration of the hospital. Hospitals also involve community members in their functions through established volunteer services. The auxiliary or volunteer group enables people from the community to make an important contribution to patient care through various types of volunteer services. The people who use the hospital's services are members of the community, and as a result their expectations of health care and services greatly influence the hospital organization. Because of this continuous community involvement in hospital services, the values of the people in the community influence the philosophy and the values adopted by the hospital organization.

Not all hospitals are community-based hospitals. The armed services hospitals, for example, are federally operated. It could be said, however, that every hospital does have a defined community of users. The Veterans Administration hospitals are used by veterans, and the armed services hospitals are used by personnel in the armed forces. In this sense, the hospital organization functions to meet its community's expectations. These hospital functions are carried out by the people who are employed by the organization. It is the function, then, of health-care professionals who are employed by the hospital to conduct the operation of the hospital in accordance with the values of the community it serves.

Professionals who are employed by hospitals have the responsibility of using the resources available in the organization to meet the unique health-care needs of the community to be served. Some of the factors that determine the unique care needs include the geographic location of the hospital, the nature of the population served, the funds available, and the number and types of other health-care agencies present in the hospital's service area. Particular patient-care needs of a population are related to the type of environmental health problems found in the location, the hazards that accompany the types of recreation and employment available in the community, and the cultural diversity and age groups within the population. Health-care needs in an urban industrial center can be quite different from those found in a rural community.

Health-care delivery system is a term used to discuss the routes through which people receive health care. While hospitals are the central core of this system, other types of health-care organizations are being developed within the health-care industry. Two types of health-care agencies of recent origin are the Neighborhood Health Centers and the Health Maintenance Organization. Public Law 89-749, which is the Public Health Service Act (section 314) passed in 1966, provided for development of federally supported health centers. These Neighborhood Health Centers are developed to meet the health-care needs of the disadvantaged and the urban poor and to provide comprehensive health services within neighborhoods. The

Health Maintenance Organization is a public, nonprofit organization designed to be self-sustaining. The Health Maintenance Act of 1973 provided for development of HMOs particularly in areas of the country where the population is medically underserved.

These types of health-care agencies are like hospitals in that they employ professionals to provide health care. They also exemplify the efforts being made to evaluate and adapt health-care agencies to the current needs of society [3]. The delivery of health-care services is a national issue, and federal legislation has been instrumental in changing health-care organizations [1]. One change is that the differentiation between private and public health-care organizations is becoming less clear. This has resulted from the use of federal and state funds by private hospitals.

Medicare and Medicaid are examples of federal and state payment for hospital services. Medicare was first legislated in amendments to the Social Security Act, Title 18, and Medicaid was legislated in amendments to the Social Security Act, Title 19, in 1965. Other examples of legislation affecting professional health-care services are Public Law 89-239, Regional Medical Programs, and Public Law 89-749, Comprehensive Health Planning, which focused on the evaluation of health-care delivery in specified regions of the country. Current legislation also includes Public Law 92-603, Professional Standards Review Organization, passed in 1972, and Public Law 93-641, the National Health Planning and Resources Development Act, both of which are concerned with health-care services. All of these legislative acts have influenced the health-care delivery system in some respects, and new legislation will continue to influence how professionals function within health-care organizations [2]. Because of this influence, professionals in the health-care field must understand how to work in and how to exert influence through their professional organizations' activity in legislation. Professionals must also exert their influence within health-care organizations.

The Role of the Professional

The professional leadership of persons in key positions in the health-care agency provides direction and interpretation of the public's expectations for service. These people "professionalize" the organization: They set the attitudes and the emotional tone for all the employees. The values of these professionals expand the values of the community in terms of the organization's philosophy. Determining priorities for patient services and establishing the working order in the organization are the responsibilities of the professionals employed by the health-care agency.

Professionals, then, determine the behaviors of employees in the organization. The implications of professionalism are important in examining how professionals determine these behaviors. Professionalism embodies making independent decisions based on specific knowledge about a defined realm of practice. Through the processes of professional education and through continued participation as members in professional organizations, professionals are ideally indoctrinated with standards and goals for practice and with a concept of ethical conduct in practice. A strong identification with a profession encourages each professional to assume a personal responsibility for fulfilling the expectations of his or her role. The professional meets these expectations through professional competence applied with integrity and pride. An organization enhances professionalism when its environment allows for the freedom to be professional and when it adheres to standards of professional behavior.

The professionals in a health-care organization represent different areas of health-care services. These persons share responsibilities for identifying common concepts and goals of patient care and for working in a cooperative manner. The organizational structure places these professionals in proximity so that they can work together. They are separated only by specialized knowledge and by specialized function. If the ideologies and personalities of professionals are compatible, the common core of knowledge about patient care can serve as the basis for intertwining of effort. If they are not compatible, there may be contention among the various professionals. The care patients receive is enhanced or hindered in accordance with the working relationships among the professionals.

In addition to the responsibilities of professionals for coordinating their work with that of other personnel who give specialized care to patients, the professionals are often expected to function with a number of subprofessionals who perform segments of their work. When professionals are assisted by others with less educational preparation to carry out a portion of their functions, they must be competent in the practice of their profession as well as in supervision of subprofessionals.

Professional nurses in hospitals, for example, are expected to be competent in giving nursing care and in directing the work of licensed practical nurses and nurse's aides. The professional nurses are the key personnel on the patient-care unit. They professionalize the organizational structure of the unit by providing a quality of patient care that is compatible with the philosophy of the hospital and with the services provided by all medical personnel. Professional nurses are assisted by persons with varying amounts of training and technical competence in patient care whose work must be supervised. The professional nurses are responsible for nursing care. What does this responsibility encompass in the total hospital organization?

It is possible for a nurse to work effectively on a patient-care unit without understanding the broad role of the nurse as part of the total hospital organization. A patient-care unit often seems complete within itself because the nurse is provided with supplies and equipment necessary for giving care and with methods of communicating with persons in other departments who are involved in a patient's care. The nurse relates most directly to the patients, to other nursing personnel, to doctors, and to all others who give direct patient care on the unit.

For this reason, nurses often perceive the hospital organization in terms of the organization of their own patient-care unit. Have you heard a nurse say, "I have never worked in a more organized hospital," because of that nurse's experiences in giving care on an organized unit in that hospital? Have you ever compared patient-care units with your friends, identifying the head nurse, the doctors, the geographic location of a unit, or the types of patient needs as causes of differences among units in a hospital? Nurses tend to evaluate the hospital through their reactions to experiences in their specific realm of practice. The patient-care unit is actually a "mini-organization" with the total hospital organization, and each of these "mini-organizations" can have its own personality and behaviors.

The personality and behaviors of the mini-organizations which make up the larger organization are a function of the behaviors of the individuals who make up the mini-organizations. Each person in the organization must be able to contribute to it in a meaningful way in order to maintain the integrity of the organization or structure. Because basic human needs are reflected through each person's individuality, his or her values and behavior determine how that individual contributes to an organizational structure.

Let us suppose that several chemicals are placed together. It is possible that the chemicals will not react. If they do, the type and degree of reaction will depend on the conditions surrounding the chemicals and the inherent characteristics of the chemicals. This is similar to placing people into an organization where continuous interaction is expected. Among typical chemical reactions (and their related people reactions) are dissociation of the chemical (conflict or confusion in people), formation of an emulsion (temporary merging of individual goals), or formation of a new product. In the new product each chemical is still identifiable through chemical analysis. However, the characteristics of the new product are different from the characteristics of the individual chemicals. In a similar way a group of people who are united to achieve a common purpose has characteristics different from those of individuals within the group.

An organization is composed of a group of people whose identities are merged into the formation of a separate entity. An analogy can be drawn between the growth and development of an organization and that of an individual. Just as each person has innate qualities and learned abilities, an organization usually grows and develops within the traditions of a community which determine what the organization is and how it ought to act in providing service. The individual's personality colors how that individual functions in society. The person has certain powers to control what he will do, where he will go, and what he will achieve. An organization has this potential for control, being different in that a group of people must activate its personality.

The relationships between the structure of the organization with its own personality and with the individual employee are crucial to the success of an organization. First of all, it is important to note that people need organizations. Human beings have a propensity for order in their relationships, which the formal organization satisfies by arranging people in a structure. People in the organizational structure are given titles and job descriptions which define the expectations of their roles. Organizational behavior evolves around these roles and expectations. Each person interprets that role in an individual manner. The differences in the way the role of a given position is interpreted reflect each person's capabilities and aptitudes. People work with others in different ways, and relationships among people are variable.

Behavior of personnel enlivens the organizational structure and is a determinant of the organization's capacity for accomplishing its purpose. The structure supports cooperation among personnel. When the personnel behave according to their defined roles, there is usually harmony within the organization. This harmony exists when employees are well matched to the expectations of their positions, when the arrangement of personnel is practical for accomplishing the work, and when pathways for communication are adequate and open.

On the other hand, discord within the structure implies that employees are not capable of meeting the expectations of their positions, that the expectations of the positions are not realistic, or that the organizational structure is not suitable for accomplishing the work. In this event the behavior of people in the organization may provide for change implementation through reevaluation of the structure and formation of a more workable order for the organization.

The behavior of all personnel is greatly influenced by the organization's philosophy. In a hospital this philosophy is basic in determining what constitutes quality patient care. Once this philosophy is defined it must be implemented by the employees in a way that best utilizes time, supplies, equipment, and human effort. To be successful in giving patient care as a group, all employees must share the same philosophy of care and common organizational objectives so that they can coordinate their efforts to achieve a common purpose.

Professionals have a major responsibility for the hospital organization's effectiveness. Because patients often perceive the hospital organization through their experiences on a patient-care unit, professional nurses are key persons among medical professionals. The continuous care provided by nurses is, for the patient, the hub of all activity in the hospital. The processes of management are used by nurses to promote their effectiveness as participants in giving health care. Nurses must be concerned about the functions of the total health-care organization and must relate in a constructive way to other medical professionals through the mechanisms of organized health services. All the work that nurses accomplish in the nursing-practice department, and more specifically on a patient-care unit, must complement that accomplished in the entire hospital. Nurses must accept the professional commitment of becoming effective managers of health care, and they must contribute to the evolution of health care through application of their professional standards and expertise.

Organizational Structure

An organizational structure is similar to the structure of the body and, as such, provides a rational design for the complexities of its function. The nurse contributes to and uses the resources of the organization and also functions within the context of the organization. In this section some concepts about organizational structures of health-care agencies are discussed to give you a perspective about how you, as a nurse, relate to an organization.

There are many similarities that can be drawn between an individual nurse and a given health-care organization. A nurse, for example, has a value system and a philosophy. An organization forms an entity that also has a value system and a philosophy. Both the individual nurse and the organization have legitimate authority to provide patient care. The nurse has a license to practice issued by the state, and the organization is a corporation with a charter outlining its purposes and functions that is granted by the state. In a sense, an organization is an aggregate of components that make up the entity just as a person is an aggregate of body systems. Both have a "personality" and function through interaction of all components. The total result of this interactive function is greater than the function of the sum of all components, a phenomenon referred to as synergy.

The organizational structure of a health-care agency reflects its value system, its philosophy, and its particular needs to function. Nursing activities are coordinated with those of other employees through the structural design of the organization. These employees can be classified as (1) those who manage the overall organization to ensure that it carries out its mission, (2) those who carry out the processes of the function of the organization, (3) those who provide the necessities for the environment in which the processes take place, and (4) those who carry out the activities necessary to maintain the organization as an entity in the community. These classifications are not clear-cut since there is overlapping among the roles of personnel in all groups. The classification is useful, however, in examining the complexities of an organization.

The people who "manage" the organization are the administrators, the department heads, and the people who are concerned with the broad and general mission of the health-care agency in its community. Those who carry out the processes of the organization's function are the health-care providers: the nurses, doctors, dietitians, and all who relate directly to the patients. People who provide the environmental requisites are those concerned with personnel functions, those who maintain the physical plant, such as engineers and housekeepers, and those who take care of the financial aspects of the agency, such as accountants and computer specialists. The organization is maintained as an entity by those people whose activities are centered on planning, development, marketing, public relations, and other such functions. These people ensure that the organization continues to have a source of clients, funds, and community support. Often these "maintenance" functions are carried out by the administrators in smaller organizations.

You can understand how complex an organization can be from the descriptions of the varied types of personnel who are employed in it. There are many different ways to organize people into an organizational structure. A hospital, for example may use a combination of structural designs to achieve its purposes. The interaction in a hospital is complex, and it is necessary to develop a rational order of relationships to ensure that the efforts of the people are efficient in carrying out the hospital's functions. Since the functions of employees are unique to their specific departments, the type of organizational structure that is appropriate for one department may not be suitable for another. The concept that form, or structure, should follow function is applied when planning the organizational structure for different departments.

There are several different models of organizational structures that have evolved from theories about how people can best be organized. The traditional model is called a bureaucratic model. Many of the theories concerning the bureaucratic model stem from the work of Max Weber [4], who perceived that an organizational structure should stabilize and clarify relationships among people in an orderly way. Among his principles of organizing are that there should be division of labor with specialization of function; that there should be a hierarchy in the arrangement of positions to provide for a flow of authority and control; that rules should be systematized to provide for uniformity and continuity and to ensure stability and coordination of effort; that relationships among people should be impersonal; and that technical competence should be provided for in the organization.

The bureaucratic plan for arranging people according to their responsibilities for doing the work of the organization can be illustrated by an organizational chart of a hospital.

TRADITIONAL ORGANIZATION—CHAIN OF RESPONSIBILITY

This chart (see p. 6) represents a traditional organization in which the chain of authority and responsibility is passed down from the board of directors to the hospital administrator and from the administrator to department heads. In classic management theories the lines formed by the diagram are referred to as the "scalar chain," illustrating the divisions of responsibility from the broad total responsibility of the administrator to the specific responsibility of personnel in a given department. As one traces the chain downward, the responsibilities of personnel become increasingly more specific. The functions of those at the top of the chain are broad functions that relate to the total organization, and the functions of those downward become increasingly delineated to a specific part of the total organization.

In traditional organizational theory, the concept of responsibility is closely aligned with three other concepts: authority, delegation, and accountability. Authority is vested in the board of directors, who in turn delegate authority to the chief executive officer, who delegates authority to the administrative staff, and so on down the line of the scalar chain. Responsibility must be accepted by the person who fills each position along the line of the scalar chain according to the functions delineated in the description of that position. Since a person cannot fulfill a given area of responsibility without authority to do so, it is necessary that authority be delegated along with the responsibilities of the position.

Authority and responsibility flow downward along the scalar chain while accountability flows upward. Accountability is a concomitant of authority which means that a person is accountable only for those functions for which he or she has the authority. When a person accepts the authority and responsibility for a position as delegated, that person is accountable for fulfilling the responsibility to those who delegate it. This statement implies that the person is not only accountable for accomplishing the work that has been delegated in such a way that the organization's goals are met, but is also responsible for the means used to achieve those goals or outcomes. A person becomes responsible for the position functions delineated by the organization when he or she accepts the position. Job descriptions that outline these functions are developed within organizations to communicate the expectation to the person who accepts the position. Job descriptions are formal statements of the functions of a given position in the organization.

Even when there are formal written job descriptions, however, the responsibilities of personnel in an organization are not always clearly defined. In some instances the formal and written descriptions lack specificity either because the position is not described well or because it is evolutionary and cannot be described with specificity. In other instances the interpretation of job descriptions changes over time as professional practices change. Professional judgment is essential in functioning in an organization because human interaction and the complexities of organizational interaction defy explicit statements of function for every aspect of position responsibilities. Knowledge and common sense are two components of professional judgment that are learned in the processes of becoming professional during one's educational experiences as well as in one's work experiences.

The scalar chain serves then to establish working relationships among personnel, while position descriptions delineate functions more specifically. An example of how a scalar chain works can be drawn from any type of organization. A department head, for example, cannot possibly fill all of the functions for the entire department. The department head delegates functions to others who accept the responsibility for performing the functions. The person who accepts the responsibility has concomitant authority and is accountable to the person who has delegated the functions.

Persons at the top of the scalar chain are responsible and accountable for functions that take place in the entire organization; the department head is responsible and accountable for functions of the department; staff members are responsible and accountable for specific functions of their positions, such as nursing care, laboratory analysis, or supply delivery. Because functions are delineated with increasing specificity downward along the chain, the phrase, "That's not my responsibility" is commonly used. You may have used this phrase yourself, and when you used it you were saying, "I do not have the authority to make that decision or to perform that function."

In addition to outlining the scalar chain, the organizational chart also serves as a guide for understanding the plan for formal communication among personnel in an organization. Channels of communication usually follow the lines of responsibility. For example, the staff nurse goes through vertical channels when communicating with the head nurse. Communication is a vital link among persons who are involved in the work to coordinate the efforts of personnel. The lines of communication in an organization are clarified by job descriptions that outline the area of responsibility and authority for each position as well as lines of communication and accountability. When all the job descriptions for employees in an organization are viewed together, it is possible to realize how each person contributes to the total organization to accomplish the work.

Although organizational structures vary among health-care agencies, each one contains provision for authority, responsibility, and accountability. A pertinent question at this point is, How does a given health-care agency arrive at its particular organizational structure? The major components that influence choice of structure include the work to be accomplished, the supplies and equipment required, the physical plant in which the work is done, the competencies of the people who do the work, and the geographic location of the physical facilities. All these components must be organized in a health-care agency so that patients receive effective, efficient, and economical care.

In a traditional hospital organization (see p. 6) the work is usually divided according to function. Departments are formed for provision of services, such as the laboratory department, the x-ray department, the surgical department, and the outpatient department. Personnel responsible for carrying out similar specialized functions are placed in a single department. In this way the physical facility can be planned to augment the work of the department, equipment and supplies can be centrally located, and communication among personnel with similar functions is facilitated. The chain of authority, responsibility, and accountability extends from the administrator down to the personnel of each specialized department through department heads.

One of the concerns in designing organizational structures is delegation of authority and responsibility. In general, authority and responsibility are delegated to the level in the organization where decisions most influence the people at that level. Decisions that are limited in their effect to a given department, for example, are made in that department, while decisions that affect the entire health-care agency are made at the administrative level. An organization can be centralized or decentralized. A centralized organization is a "tall" organizational design in which the locus of decision-making is placed centrally at the top of the organization. A decentralized organization is a "flat" design in which the locus for decision-making is disseminated to various departments or units.

In a decentralized organization, more decision-making authority and responsibility, and thus more control, is delegated throughout the structure. To be effective, a decentralized organization requires that decision-makers be competent since important organizational decisions are made at various divisions in the organization. The advantage is that people in the various decentralized units of the organization can adapt to changes more readily because they make decisions at a local level. A centralized organization provides for stability and uniformity throughout the entire organization since the locus of decision-making and control is found at the level of the organizational hierarchy. In a centralized structure, decisions are made more slowly because more time is required for communication to pass to and from the decision-makers. A typical bureaucratic structure is a tall, centralized organization.

SYSTEMS AND MATRIX ORGANIZATIONAL STRUCTURES

The *systems approach* is another type of organizational design. In this design, communication flows horizontally and laterally, and there is more flexibility in decision-making than in a centralized, traditional organizational structure. Some theorists believe that most health-care agency organizations are actually open systems because there is a continuous flow of input from patients, families, professional groups, community groups, public policy, and state and federal legislation.

Theoretically, a system is composed of feedback loops including input into the system, transformation processes that take place within the system, output from the system, and feedback that influences the input into the system. One basic concept of systems is that of equifinality, which means that goals or values can be attained through a number of different paths or means. The system remains in equilibrium until some factor of input or of the transformation processes, called throughput, changes. The system adapts to changes and can be responsive to them because of the greater flexibility in decision-making.

In a systems approach, the patient, with individual needs and capabilities, is a source of input that becomes part of the system. The patient goes through the system according to his or her individual needs, using only those components or subsets of the system required for care. A physician or a nurse-practitioner routes the patient through the system, determining the pathway the patient should take according to the assessment of the patient's needs and the patient's wishes to participate in the diagnosis, care, or treatment processes. The subsets of the system are different specialized services such as x-ray, surgery, or diet therapy, and all of these subsets are integrated in the system to provide patient care. The cycle of events in the care of any given patient is individualized, and the patient is the focus of all of the services provided.

Yet another type of organizational structure is the *matrix organization*. The matrix organization is a group of mini-organizations within a larger organizational structure. There may be a skeleton of a traditional hierarchical structure, but there is no well-defined scalar chain with its unity of command and clear delegation of authority and responsibility. Instead, people are arranged according to specialized processes or functions, and are responsible and accountable for managing these functions more autonomously than in a traditional bureaucratic structure. Communication flows in all directions: upward, downward, horizontally, and laterally. People communicate with others in the organization according to their needs for the use of resources or the functions of others. This direct communication among employees emphasizes the interaction processes among people rather than the structural design for communication designated by the scalar chain in traditional organizations.

For the matrix organization to be effective, the people in the organization must be secure enough and competent enough to assert themselves and to negotiate for integration of function in the organization. This type of organizational structure works well when there is a desire or need to modify the present working relationships and products or when innovation is desired. The interaction of individuals across organizational lines provides for checks and balances. People tend to relate to one another according to their areas of specialization rather than through superior-subordinate relationships that are formed in the traditional organizational structure. Because there is no strong hierarchical structure to provide for stability, authority and responsibility are distributed throughout the organization. Checks and balances occur as people representing their mini-organizations negotiate for resources, for input from other mini-organizations, and for development of mechanisms that provide for integration of function. There is potential for conflict within matrix organizations because the behavior of employees is emphasized, rather than strong unity of command and central control. The matrix organizational structure promotes independent thinking, creativity, and collaborative relationships.

Both the systems and the matrix organizational structures are more flexible than the traditional structure, and they are appropriately used in situations where there is continual growth and change. Both provide for meeting contingencies since decision-making authority and responsibility are located at the level of "processes" in the organization.

The systems approach is excellent for focusing on the work to be accomplished, especially when many different types of activities are required for patient care. An example of the systems approach in patient care is an agency in which the patient is routed to different specialty areas. Nurses, dietitians, laboratory technicians, x-ray technicians, and social service caseworkers are subsets of the system that are integrated in giving care. Patient care is given in a composite of interrelated activities. The various medical personnel all cooperate in planning care.

Most organizations include variations of traditional and innovative structures. The nature of the work of hospitals defies a singular approach to organization of all departments. For example, the systems theories are easiest to apply when all the information about the requirements of patient care, the specifications for giving care, and the supplies and equipment necessary are well defined. All this information can be computed to determine a sequence of activities which most effectively and efficiently accomplishes the work.

However, the activities involved in giving patient care cannot be specifically described and analyzed for the inherent requirements of every patient because of the unknown element of differences in patient needs. Each patient presents an individual set of problems which cannot always be anticipated. Even though general and common needs of patients can be defined and planned for, the plans must be flexible to accommodate the individual. The matrix organization is suited to development of a flexible and responsive structure.

A matrix organization is effective in health-care agencies that are experimenting with innovations in patient-care service delivery. Mini-organizations are formed to provide specialized patient care such as crisis intervention, oncology, or cardiovascular-respiratory patient-care units. The personnel in the mini-organization form a specialized team or group to carry out the function of the unit. These personnel communicate directly with personnel in other departments, such as the laboratory department, the planning department, or the social service department. Through this direct communication they negotiate for provision of the support or resources they require to develop and maintain the mini-organization's specialized function. Each mini-organization depends on the supporting services of the total organization or macro-organization for administrative and management functions. The mini-units are different in that the services developed are unique to the types of care requisites presented by the group of patients who use the particular services.

The arrangement of people in an organization is affected by the type of work they do, by the placement of facilities in the agency, and by the patient's needs. All types of organizational structures deal with the provision of service to patients in which service is the focal point.

Organizational structures place people in a working order and depend on people to accomplish the work. Once the organizational structure is defined, the continuity of patient services depends on the behavior of the people who fill the structure.

Study Questions

1. What contribution do you, as a professional nurse, make to a health-care organization?
2. Describe the sources of legal authority that legitimize the function of the organization to provide patient care.
3. Describe how an organizational structure supports a board member's fulfillment of accountability for services provided by the health-care agency.
4. Speculate about what would happen if a department head did not accept the responsibility for patient services in the department.
5. How does an organizational structure design influence decision-making in an organization?
6. In what types of situations should a centralized organizational structure be used? A decentralized organizational structure?
7. Analyze the relationships you develop with other people in a hospital organization as a staff nurse by (a) listing the specialized functions of those that you have communicated with person-to-person, by phone only, and by requisition only; and (b) explaining how the functions of the people you have listed contribute to your patient's care.
8. Describe your expectations of a hospital organization as (a) an employee, and (b) a user of hospital services.
9. Describe how a health-care agency relates to its community. Using an agency you are familiar with as an example, explain how that agency cooperates with other organizations in the community in providing health care.

References

1. Ball, R. M. Background of Regulation in Health Care. In Institute of Medicine, *Controls in Health Care*. Washington, D.C.: National Academy of Sciences, 1975. Pp. 3–22.
2. Duval, M. K. The Provider, the Government, and the Consumer. In J. H. Knowles (ed.), *Doing Better and Feeling Worse: Health Care in the United States*. New York: W. W. Norton, 1977. Pp. 185–192.
3. Gosfield, A. *PSROs: The Law and the Health Consumer*. Cambridge: Ballinger, 1975. Pp. 1–19.
4. Henderson, A. M., and Parsons, T. (Trans. and eds.) *Max Weber: The Theory of Social and Economic Organization*. New York: The Free Press, 1947 (Copyright the Oxford University Press, New York). Pp. 329–331.

Suggested Reading

Aden, G. D. Hospitals must lead the way in meeting public's demands. *Hospitals* 51:58–61, Nov. 16, 1977.

Aspen Systems Corp. *Problems in Hospital Law* (2nd ed.). Rockville, Md.: Aspen, 1974.

Austin, C. J. Redefining professionalism in health administration. *Hosp. Prog.* 58:70–73, 97, May 1977.

Bice, T. W., and Salkever, D. S. Certificate-of-need programs: Cure or cause of inflated costs? *Hosp. Prog.* 58:65–67, 100, July 1977.

Buchele, R. B. *The Management of Business and Public Organizations.* New York: McGraw-Hill, 1977.

Colner, A. N. The impact of state government rate setting on hospital management. *Health Care Manage. Rev.* 2:37–49, Winter 1977.

Danielson, J. M. Health consortium responds to total health care needs. *Hospitals* 51:69–73, March 1, 1977.

Dessler, G. *Organization and Management: A Contingency Approach.* Englewood Cliffs, N.J.: Prentice-Hall, 1976.

Forward Plan for Health FY 1977–81, June 1975. USDHEW, PHS, DHEW Publication No. (OS) 76-50024. Washington, D.C.: U.S. Govt. Printing Office, 1975.

French, R. *The Dynamics of Health Care.* (2nd ed.). New York: McGraw-Hill, 1974.

Friedman, E. Medicaid: The primrose path. *Hospitals* 51:51–56, Aug. 16, 1977.

Friedman, E. Medicaid: A crop of nettles. *Hospitals* 51:73–80, Sept. 16, 1977.

Friedman, E. Medicaid: One seed for the crow. *Hospitals* 51:61–66, Oct. 1, 1977.

Friedman, E., and Wandorf, C. Medicaid: A garden sown with dragon's teeth. *Hospitals* 51:59–64, Sept. 1, 1977.

Greenberg, W. HMO's stimulate competition, FTC concludes. *Hosp. Prog.* 58:10–11, Oct. 1977.

Hall, V. C. *Statutory Regulation of the Scope of Nursing Practice—A Critical Survey.* Chicago: National Joint Practice Commission, 1975.

Harlow, D. N., and Hanke, J. *Behavior in Organizations.* Boston: Little, Brown, 1975.

Health Policy Making in Action: The Passage and Implementation of the National Health Planning and Resources Development Act of 1974 (Publication #41-1600). New York: National League for Nursing, 1975.

Kelly, L. Y. Credentialing of health care personnel. *Nurs. Outlook* 25:562–569, Sept. 1977.

Kirlane, M., and Grimes, P. Improving a hospital organization chart. *Hosp. Prog.* 58:85–89, Sept. 1977.

Leonard, A., and Rogers, I. Prescription for survival. *Superv. Nurse* 8:22–24, Nov. 1977.

Luthans, F. *Organizational Behavior* (2nd ed.). New York: McGraw-Hill, 1977.

Marriner, A. Adaptive organizational models. *Superv. Nurse* 8:44–50, Aug. 1977.

McLaughlin, C. P. Productivity and human services. *Health Care Manage. Rev.* 1:47–60, Fall 1976.

Monaco, R. J., and Smith, T. T. How supervisors can put systems to work in day to day management. *Hosp. Top.* 55:34, 36–41, Sept./Oct. 1977.

Prybil, L. O. Hospital boards face increasing demands. *Hospitals* 51:103–106, April 1, 1977.

Rosen, H. M., Metsch, J. M., and Levey, S. *The Consumer and the Health Care System: Social and Managerial Perspectives.* New York: Spectrum Publications, 1977.

Rosser, J. M., and Mossberg, H. E. *An Analysis of Health Care Delivery.* New York: Wiley, 1977.

Salkever, D. S., and Bice, T. W. *Impact of State Certificate-of-Need Laws on Health Care Costs and Utilization.* USDHEW PHS NCHSR Research Digest Series (HRA) 77-3163.

Schulz, R., and Johnson, A. C. *Management of Hospitals.* New York: McGraw-Hill, 1976.

Skerry, W. PL 93-641: Beyond planning toward control. *Hosp. Prog.* 57:10, 30, March 1976.

Somers, A. R., and Somers, H. M. *Health and Health Care: Policies in Perspective.* Germantown, Md.: Aspen, 1977.

Stagl, J. M. A look ahead at the forces of change. *Hospitals* 51:74–78, March 16, 1977.

Swanburg, R. C. *Management of Patient Care Services.* St. Louis: Mosby, 1976.

2. The Role of the Manager

What does a manager do? In order to answer this question, one must first answer some other basic questions. What is management? Are managers necessary? How do managers function in an organization? In the previous chapter we considered organizations, the general role of a professional in an organization, and organizational structures. This chapter is concerned with the role of the manager and with management processes. As you study these general management processes, consider your own concept of management.

The Concept and Processes of Management

During your life, you have had many experiences with management. You have belonged to organizations: a school, a church, or a youth club. Your experiences in these organizations have influenced your present concept of management. In addition to your experiences in organized groups, you have probably been a manager in many situations, since management is an integral part of human life. Have you ever managed something? Have you ever been managed? How did this management take place? In answering these questions, you will find that you already have a frame of reference about management. As you expand this frame of reference in the study of nursing management, you will find that your past experiences and your common sense are valuable assets in assuming a management role in nursing.

ELEMENTS OF MANAGEMENT

Chester Bernard [1] has written that organizations are social systems. Using this theory as a basis for management, you can view the role of the manager as working effectively within a social system to accomplish goals. Management processes such as organizing, activating, controlling, and evaluating are used to accomplish organizational goals. Underlying each of these processes are two major requisites in all management processes, communication and decision-making. The quality of the communication and of the decision-making is further undergirded by the manager's knowledge and conceptual ability.

Management is a composite of many interrelated components. The manager's personal attributes and capabilities affect how management processes are used. The management processes are techniques

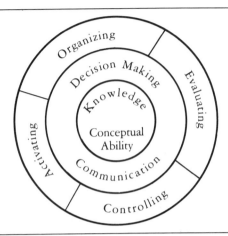

to be used in the perspective of the environment, the organizational goals, and the specific nature of the goals and objectives in the manager's realm of function, which in nursing management is patient care. Management techniques provide ways of dealing with the variable factors involved in achieving purposes, such as people's ideas and efforts, clients' needs, equipment, supplies, and the workplace itself. The manager's personal interpretation of situations and events and the manager's personal characteristics affect the way that the manager will use these management processes in bringing a sense of order to the integration of the variable factors inherent in accomplishing the work.

Management is an evolving field of study, and theories of management are being developed continually through observation and research. Just as nursing has a body of knowledge with specific terminology, management has its own body of knowledge and related terminology. Because management can mean different things to different people, the meanings of words and the interpretations of concepts can be confusing to one who is just beginning to study management. To develop a sense of management concepts and to facilitate communication about management, it is useful to develop a framework of thought about management processes. This framework can provide you with a mechanism for studying about management and for analyzing your own concept of management.

MAJOR MANAGEMENT PROCESSES
For our purposes in developing such a framework, let us consider that management includes four major processes: organizing, activat-

ing, controlling, and evaluating. These processes are interrelated and sometimes overlap. They are also continuous processes that extend throughout all management functions. The purposes of an organization are accomplished through management processes that bring people, supplies, equipment, and other resources together in an orderly way to perform a service or to create a product. In performing the desired service or creating the designated product, changes take place through the behavior of people as they use their ideas, knowledge, equipment, supplies, and facilities. The manager's role is to ensure that all of the necessary elements for performing the service or for producing the product are available, usable, appropriate, and maintained and that the efforts or behaviors of people are effective in the performance of the work roles that bring about the changes necessary to provide the service or to create the product.

Organizing. Organizing is an initial management process that takes place before the work is begun. It is also a continuous process that takes place as the work is being accomplished because portions of any activity are continuously organized in view of new information or new developments in any given situation. When organizing, the manager determines a plan that outlines the work to be accomplished, who should do the work, how they should accomplish the work, when the work should be carried out, and what materials or resources are required. The plan is based on an overall determination of a goal or of expected outcomes.

Organizing, then, is determining how the pieces of an activity can be arranged into interlocking sections. The manager's philosophy about the work, conceptual ability, and decision-making ability influence how people, places, and things are placed together as interlocking sections to achieve the determined goals. The manager forms a concept of the activities to be accomplished, sets standards for methods to be used according to his or her philosophy and knowledge of the prerequisites of the activities, and uses decision-making processes in determining how to arrange all of the components in an order that will both satisfy the standards for performance and achieve the desired outcomes.

Activating. Activating is the process of giving life to the plans made in organizing; it is a dynamic process of "making things happen." When plans are implemented in the work situation, people are performing the "processes" inherent in their functions. Activating emphasizes the human relations aspect of management, particularly in health-care agencies, which are labor-intensive organizations. Some of the components of activating are making sure that people understand the expectations set forth in the plans, gaining the workers' acceptance of authority and responsibility, fostering their motivation to perform and to perform well, guiding people in personal growth through work experiences, directing the work, supporting the workers as they deal with the challenges and problems of their work, and supervising and coordinating all of the elements or inputs as necessary to accomplish the work.

The process of activating requires continual decision-making about people, places, and things to enable the manager to adapt to situations that occur and to accommodate the plans to the realistic working situation. Plans made in the organizing phase provide a frame of reference for these decisions. They also specify the general direction that the manager pursues in making decisions, so that consistency can be maintained. This consistency is a factor in establishing effective working relationships in the processes of carrying out the work and also in maintaining a perspective about the desired end results.

Controlling. Controlling includes aspects of both organizing and activating. The plans made in organizing are the basis for control, and the way that the plans are implemented in the activating phase affects the outcomes achieved. Control can be interpreted as providing stability and maintaining the work environment. Controlling is closely associated with activating since it comprises such activities as supervising, measuring performance, assessing situations, making decisions about changes that should be made in plans, and ensuring that people have the requisites necessary for their work. Controlling must take into account unforeseen problems or events, such as lack of planned resources, illness of an employee, or changes in external events, that have an impact on the activity being managed.

The essence of the process of controlling is manipulating the environment to create a desirable work situation and making sure that the workers meet the prescribed standards. This involves providing people with an environment conducive to work—one in which they may realize their potential by accomplishing the work in an appropriate manner that is satisfying to them. Controlling involves providing adequate time and sufficient supplies, equipment, and resources to do the work. Controlling also means providing sufficient structure so that the behavior of the workers is focused on the work to be accomplished. Controlling is complex in that the processes of controlling are integral to every organizational activity. The manager who wishes to develop employees through work relationships can foster growth and participation by controlling the environment, the modes of interaction, the assignment of functions, and the information the employees receive about their work. That type of control frees the employees to develop and to grow in their work. When the organizational structure facilitates positive working relationships by formalizing job descriptions, for example, the job descriptions serve to "control" human activities.

Often the word control is associated with limit-setting and disciplinary action. Both are aspects of control that must be used by the manager. When the manager exerts control in the form of discipline, the manager is limiting the employee's behaviors to those acceptable to the organization. Such disciplinary action is most successful if other aspects of the organization are controlled in the positive sense by clearly defining functions, roles, and responsibilities that must be met by employees, and by providing the necessary requisites for effectively carrying out the work. The way one "activates" work in the organization is an integral part of the control process. Leadership and group interaction, both of which are discussed in a later chapter, are management behaviors applied in the activating of organizational work and both impact on a given manager's use of control processes.

Evaluating. Evaluating is also generally applicable to each management process; evaluating is planned for in the organizing process, is a component of the activating process, and both provide input and uses feedback from the controlling process. Standards determined in the organizing process are the criteria for evaluating. These standards include those that apply to the process of the work and those that apply to the outcomes. They are compared not only to what actually happens while the work is being performed, but also to the end results. The results of these comparisons are called feedback, and this feedback is used to determine new and better ways to organize the work.

Decision-making is an integral part of the evaluation process. The manager determines standards through decision-making and also makes decisions about what to measure and about how to measure performance. Decisions are also made about the types of tools that are developed to measure the qualitative and quantitative aspects of any activity. The feedback made available to the manager through evaluation processes must be interpreted. For example, when desired results are not achieved, the manager must decide whether the initial goals are realistic, whether the number or type of employees is appropriate to accomplish the work, whether different or new materials should be used, or whether new procedures or performance standards should be developed. The manager has to achieve a balance in developing controls that are sufficient to provide for stability, but that are not limiting or restrictive of performance, and this balance is determined through evaluation. The manager also has to develop continually evaluation tools that are valid and reliable in providing feedback.

Relationship of Managers to the Organization

The management processes are implemented by managers to ensure that customers receive the desired services or products. In so doing, the management processes also focus on ensuring that workers receive guidance, support, and a sense of satisfaction from their work. In a health-care agency it is imperative that patients receive the best quality of care possible for the money spent. The employees are essential to the quality of patient care, and it is necessary that these employees experience a sense of satisfaction in their work because productivity is a corollary of job satisfaction.

Management of groups of people for achieving a purpose within an organization is a social process. Managers must provide for a state of equilibrium in which the workers' needs are satisfied while the organization achieves its purposes. This requires that incentives provided for the workers be as great as the contributions they are expected to make to the organization. The manager is also an employee of the organization and meets personal needs through work. In an organization, the manager functions within a structure and is supported by the structure. The manager contributes his or her own talents and resources to the organization and in return receives benefits from the organization. The relationship between the manager and the organization can be complementary.

ROLE CONFLICTS IN THE ORGANIZATION

A complementary relationship between a manager and an organization is the product of many factors. One basic factor is the similarity between the manager's expectation of his role and the organization's expectation of the manager's role. Getzels and Guba [2] have defined a theoretical formula of different types of role conflicts that may occur. In addition to the potential for role conflict between the manager and the organization, there is also the potential for conflict between the role expectations of employment and the person's individual needs (role-personality conflict). While there are other sources of role conflict, these two have been selected for discussion in this chapter because they are commonly experienced by beginning managers.

Not all organizations are alike in behaviors. Some organizations are highly structured and tend to be closed, whereas others are more flexible and tend to be open. When a manager works in an organization, the scope and depth of his or her use of management processes is determined to some extent by the latitude allowed by the organization and to some extent by the manager's capabilities of expressing his or her personality. The effectiveness of a manager in any organization is relative to the relationship developed by the manager with the organization. When the manager's expectations are well matched to the organization's expectations of the managerial role, the manager will probably be effective. When there is dissonance between the manager's expectations and those of the organization, conflict can result and the manager may not be effective.

The other source of role conflict mentioned is the role-personality conflict. The manager accepts authority and responsibility for the managerial role and implements management processes to achieve work. When the manager's needs conflict with these role expectations, the manager may not be effective. This person may have difficulty working within the organizational structure and may have problems in communicating and in decision-making because of the conflict between personal needs and organizational goals.

A third source of potential conflict that exists between managers and organizations is professional role conflict. The professional brings an identity to the role of management that is distinct from the organization's structure and functions. Professionals are generally expected to initiate and follow through with implementation of management processes that are designed to meet professional standards. These professional standards are "cosmopolitan," that is, they are universally shared by the profession on a state or national basis. The professional may find that a given organization has local standards that conflict with the cosmopolitan standards. The potential for this type of conflict is great in hospitals since they tend to be stable organizational structures that change slowly. The profession of nursing is changing continually, and role expectations of the professionals have the potential for changing more rapidly than the organization's role expectations for those professionals. The nurse-manager should be aware of the values and attitudes held by the organization about nursing functions and roles. Because the professionals are accountable for maintaining a standard of practice, they are responsible for interpreting these standards to others in the organization.

Managerial Characteristics

The manager uses the processes of management to accomplish work and to ensure that this work meets professional standards. Through effective use of these processes of management, it is possible to demonstrate how these professional standards benefit the organization. The nurse-manager's capability for interpreting nursing to the organization and for prudently implementing management processes that "actualize" nursing in the organization is a major factor in producing effective management in a particular organization. The manager greatly influences the organization, as is demonstrated by variations in the way that different head nurses in a given health-care agency manage their patient-care units. The manager can be viewed as a liaison person who sets the tone for the nature of work relationships among personnel and the organization. Therefore, the manager's personal contribution is a very important aspect of organizational behavior.

What types of people make the best managers? This question is difficult to answer since different situations require different types of managers. In general, one could speculate that a self-actualized person will be a good manager. Shostrom's theory of self-actualization [3] is applicable to an examination of positive managerial characteristics. Shostrom has based much of his work on Maslow's theories of human needs (Chap. 6) and explains self-actualization as congruence between a person's inner core and his or her facade. The inner core is said to be the person's essential nature, and the facade is the person's public behavior. Some of the characteristics important in the communication functions of a manager are also characteristics of a self-actualized person.

Shostrom describes the self-actualized person as one who is capable of trust, is flexible, and has the ability to be responsive and open. He says that this person has a "permeable skin" that enables him or her to absorb new ideas and points of view. The self-actualized person is also expressive, being able to communicate inner feelings and perceptions effectively, whether they be positive or negative. In describing the less actualized person, Shostrom uses the words "less trusting, more rigid, more controlling, more manipulative, and more concerned with impressing others than with expressing core feelings and perceptions." The less actualized person tends to be defensive and resistant. Shostrom views self-actualization as a lifelong process in which the person strives continually to reach a state of congruence between individual core feelings and perceptions and the external facade of behavior. The effective manager is also growth-oriented in the continual effort to develop realistic perceptions of role, function, and organizational goals and to deal openly and rationally with problems and conflicts that arise in implementing management processes.

The Manager's Relationship to the Organization

The nurse is primarily involved in managing patient care, and, nursing functions require support of many different types of personnel employed by a health-care agency. This means that in addition to relating to the nursing staff and to patients, the nurse must relate to numbers of other personnel. Some of these relationships are based on the dependence of nurses on departments which provide supplies, equipment, and services. Others are based on the need to coordinate patient care with services provided by specialized departments such as dietary, social service, and occupational therapy.

The complexity of integrating the activities of all these personnel is illustrated by the following comments from a patient:

I hadn't been feeling well for quite some time so my doctor finally talked me into going to the hospital for some tests. This is the first time I've been in a hospital as a patient. I didn't realize how confusing it could be! It is difficult to get to know what people are supposed to do for you. Why, I've been here for just twenty-four hours and just listen to my account of the number of people I've met already.

First there was the admissions clerk, then the orderly who brought me to this room. After I was shown about by the nurse's aide, who also took my temperature, I was interviewed by the charge nurse—I think it was the head nurse. Then my doctor came in, and after he left I was examined by a resident and two interns—separately and in rapid succession. Finally it was time for dinner and another man brought in the tray. After dinner someone came in and asked me if I wanted a newspaper. That was the ward clerk. Two nurses came in to prepare me for sleep—one made the bed and the other gave me some pills. That was after someone gave me an enema or two.

The next morning I woke up and watched the housekeeping man clean the hall outside my room. There wasn't any breakfast. Instead I talked with the laboratory technician who took some blood, and then I was taken to the x-ray department by a fellow who said he was from the transfer department. In x-ray I met two technicians and a doctor who was in charge of my x-rays. Since I've been back in my room, I've seen another man with a breakfast tray, I've talked with the volunteer who checked my menu for tomorrow, to someone from accounting about my insurance number, and to the man who came in to fix the window shade. Now you are making my bed. I just wonder who keeps all these people straight? How do you know what is going on?

Integration by Organizational Control

This patient perceives an organization as a complex intermingling of people. The nurse perceives the total organization through the perspective of direct patient care. As one becomes increasingly involved in management, the interrelatedness of various departments becomes more obvious. The organization provides for integration of the many departments through organizational plans that assure employees stability, support, and routes and methods for communication.

STABILITY

Stability for employees means that the working environment is orderly and efficient. For nurses it means that linen is delivered to the patient-care unit, that special diets are prepared and delivered to patients, that someone is available to repair broken beds and other equipment, and that medications are available when patients need them. It also means that employees know where to obtain information, how to request supplies and services, and how to procure equipment.

For the nurse, efficient care depends on these services. Consider how your efficiency would be affected if you had to spend an hour to procure linen for a patient's bed or if you had to wait two days to get a bed repaired. What do you do if the patient wants his hair cut, a book to read, or a comb? Where do you get information about the insurance plan that your patient is so worried about?

SUPPORT

Supporting services provide stability by freeing the nurse to make alterations and adaptations when providing patient care. Patient care is dynamic; patient needs are constantly changing. Nurses are better able to cope with changes if their environment is orderly.

In addition to supporting employees through services, the organization supports them through policies and procedures which guide decision-making. If the hospital policy states that all patients must have a CBC, a chest x-ray, a urinalysis, and a physical examination before a surgical operation, the nurse can make the decision that a patient be retained in his room until these tests have been performed. The policy gives the nurse security because it applies equally to the actions of the doctor, the x-ray technician, the laboratory technician, and the operating room personnel. All employees must comply with this policy unless there is good reason for an exception.

COMMUNICATION

Communication serves to integrate the work of employees by facilitating both the sharing and developing of ideas and the exchange of information and requests. The scope of communication ranges from automatic and specific communication to complex discussion. Specific communications include orders for supplies, requests for services, and reports that provide information. Requisitions for laboratory work and forms for daily reports are examples of automatic methods for communication. Meetings, conferences, and channels of communication are often made routine so that employees whose activities are interrelated communicate regularly. Just as a group of staff nurses requires communication, the groups of employees representative of all departments must communicate for coordination of efforts.

In order to provide stability for coordinated function, organizations have designed plans to integrate behaviors of employees. These plans are often referred to as standard operating policies, procedures, and rules. Organizations also require developmental planning, which is necessary for the perpetuation of the organization in a changing society. An organization must project its goals to the future to ensure that it will be able to accommodate readily to changing needs of clients and to maintain its level of goal achievement.

Standard or integrating plans provide for consistent interaction among employees. Developmental plans, in contrast, provide for change implementation. The integrating plans are geared to day-by-day operations and are often the result of developmental planning which brings about changes in these day-by-day operations. Developmental plans are either short-range or long-range. Short-range plans may meet the needs of the organization for periods of months while long-range plans may encompass periods of three to five years or more. Developmental plans are visionary in nature and are future oriented.

Both integrating and developmental plans are necessary for organizing, activating, controlling, and evaluating the work of an organization over time. You may be more familiar with standard integrating plans because of your short-term experiences with organizations. When you work in an organization for a short period of time, you learn how to work within that organization by following the integrating plans in carrying out your functions. When you assume a long-term position in an organization you can better perceive the differences between the integrating plans that guide your function and the developmental plans that are focused on change implementation.

When you assume a management position, you continually evaluate the effectiveness of the integrating plans in the day-by-day operations. As organizational functions change through new developments in technology, new definition of roles, or better delineation of patient-care measures, the integrating plans must be changed to accommodate new requirements for coordinating work. Some integrating plans become obsolete with the introduction of new technology or new methods of giving care. Developments in patient care, such as checking patient's blood pressure at every clinic visit as a part of risk management, may change the integrating plans. In some instances, new integrating plans are developed to ensure the successful application of changes in function.

The purpose of developmental planning is to devise better ways of providing services or to determine how the organizational functions can be changed to meet new needs. Legislation that creates new regulations, cost containment activities, and other types of external influences may create the need for developmental planning to determine how the functions of staff can be changed so that the regulations or constraints can be met while also accomplishing the organization's mission. The purposes, goals, and objectives of any activity, the types of materials and supplies needed, and the mechanisms for interaction among personnel for carrying out newly defined functions are accomplished by developmental planning. Integrating plans emerge from developmental plans as requisites established for stability in use of organizational resources.

Integrative Plans

Organizations have established integrative plans which guide personnel in working together. These include written and unwritten statements of policy, procedures, and rules. However, each organization differs in how it expects employees to work together. Norms of organizational behavior are established according to each situation. Integrative plans serve to stabilize the environment, to support personnel, and to provide for communication. Managers from all departments are involved in using these integrative plans; the nurse-manager is no exception.

COMPONENTS OF INTEGRATIVE PLANS

Integrative plans may be said to have three components: a concept, a procedure, and specific criteria that are crucial to successful results. These components are inherent requisites of all policies, procedures, and rules. A brief definition of each will clarify their purposes in the organization.

A *concept* is a broad general statement that is derived from the health-care agency's philosophy. *Policies* are most representative of statements of concepts. These serve to influence decisions made by personnel in all departments so that their work is focused continually on the agency's goals. Concepts serve as a guide for definition of procedures and rules.

A *procedure* is a guide to performance of an activity. Procedures may be very general or specific, depending on the complexity of the activity being performed and the capabilities of the personnel who use the procedure. Procedures are written in sufficient detail to provide the information required by all persons who are involved in the activity. Task structure, through specific and detailed procedural guides for performance of activities, is needed by personnel with less experience and education. Procedures include a statement of purpose, designation of who is to perform the activity, listing of supplies and equipment required, recommendation for methods or routes of communication, and criteria for performance.

Specific criteria that are crucial to successful results are usually stated as *rules*. These rules are single-purpose statements that define what must be done or what should not be done. Consider the rule: Personnel must wear masks in the surgical suite. This is an important rule that deals with only one of a composite of activities related to maintaining asepsis in the surgical suite. Rules are clear-cut and are designed to help personnel form habits which are conducive to good practice. Policies, procedures, and rules may be written for activities that involve every department or for activities that are specific to a given department. Generally they form a continuum of general to specific guides to action, the policy being the most general. Policies that affect every department may be interpreted in procedures that are different according to a given department's responsibilities for performing an activity. In this case each department's procedures relate to the overall policy in such a way that everyone involved is working toward accomplishment of the same general purpose.

Policies, procedures, and rules may be unwritten in an organization. In this situation they are often passed along among employees by word of mouth. Unwritten policies, procedures, and rules are learned through an acculturation process when a new employee begins to work in an organization. Such bits of advice as "Always have a stethoscope when you work on 5 West because Mrs. Hill, the head nurse, does not like to see nurses without them," reflect an unwritten rule. Unwritten plans usually develop from personal preferences of managers or from accepted ways of doing things that have proved to be successful for employees. Sometimes they embellish the written policies, procedures, and rules and sometimes they contradict them. Unless the written plans are consistently enforced, the unwritten plans take precedence.

The interrelatedness of departmental functions is demonstrated by a hospital policy concerning admission of patients. The policy states that hospital beds must be kept available for admission of patients with emergency illnesses. This policy is interpreted by the admissions department and the emergency room. A procedure might be written to define the priority needs of patients that make them eligible for admission to reserved emergency beds. The procedure might be developed from guidelines established in the admissions department or the emergency room through practice. These guidelines may formalize previously unwritten procedures for those departments.

The nursing department may also have a procedure relating to this policy that might specify which personnel and which units are assigned to care for patients with emergency conditions. Another department that might be affected by the same policy is the housekeeping department. This department's related procedure may specify that three beds must always be available in the event that a patient must be temporarily placed in a lounge or a hallway when all regular hospital beds are full.

MANUALS OF POLICY AND PROCEDURE

How does a nurse find out about the written organizational policies, procedures, or rules? There are various methods that can be used to inform personnel of organizational expectations. Most hospitals, for example, have a manual of operating policies, procedures, or both. This manual includes information about many aspects of patient care, such as admission and discharge of patients. Requirements of the hospital concerning medical records, transfer of patients, consulting services, and special care units can often be found in the operating policy manual. Some statements written for manuals are broad and serve to guide decision-making by personnel. Others specify the procedure to be followed in performing a sequence of related activities.

Specific and Nonspecific Policies. Consider two statements concerning admission of patients to a convalescent care unit. The first states: Patients who require extended care services for rehabilitation through occupational and physical therapy will be admitted to the extended care unit. The second states: Transfer of patients to the extended care unit must first be approved by the committee for continuity of care. The committee consists of a physiatrist as chairman, two medical doctors, two nurses, an occupational therapist, a physical therapist, and a social caseworker. Requests for approval must be submitted to this committee on form #276. All questions concerning prognosis, care requirements, and plans for future care must be answered in their entirety by the physician or head nurse.

The first statement is a broad policy that can be interpreted in different ways by different people. Rehabilitation has many meanings, and thus the rationale for admitting patients to the extended care unit may include a variety of factors. Referring personnel need only justify the patient's need for rehabilitation by indicating that the patient requires physical and occupational therapy. The second statement, however, is outlined in more detail. Interpretation of the procedure is limited to members of the specified committee. Both statements provide information about the operation of the hospital and influence decisions that are made by persons related to the patient's care.

Departmental Policy Manuals. In addition to the general policy manual, which specifies concepts and procedures of care for all employees, various departments in the organization may have their own policy or procedure manuals. Among these are the x-ray, laboratory, personnel, and nursing departments.

Departmental policy and procedure manuals serve many functions. They can be used to inform personnel of procedures that should be observed, as a review of activities involved in performance of certain tasks or techniques, for orientation of new personnel, for teaching subprofessional employees, and for communication among personnel from different departments who perform related functions. For example, the nurse can determine how to prepare a patient for a laboratory test by reading about the test in the laboratory department's procedure manual.

Regulations and the Nurse-Manager

How does the nurse-manager become involved in policies, procedures, and rules? First of all, the nurse should understand the purpose of all these plans. Policies, procedures, and rules are organizing plans that direct and coordinate activities of all employees. When managers in each department observe these plans, they are supporting the hospital's goals to provide efficient, orderly, and safe performance.

Secondly, the nurse-manager should be well-informed about the policies, procedures, and rules, because the manager is expected to set an example by observing them. The manager's role also includes interpreting and clarifying policies, procedures, and rules and consistently enforcing them. Information, interpretation, and clarification are basic to effective enforcement. Cooperation of staff members is augmented if they understand the relationships of procedures and rules to the concepts from which they are derived.

Next, the manager is expected to evaluate the effectiveness of the policies, procedures, and rules with respect to their purposes. This is particularly true for procedures and rules. Because following procedures and rules falls into the realm of habitual activity, personnel sometimes become so accustomed to a rule that they cease to evaluate its usefulness in achieving the intended purpose. This may result in perpetuation of an activity long after the need for it has diminished because of changes in the related concept.

Nurses are primarily concerned with integrative behaviors directly related to provision of patient care, and this requires using procedures such as standard order forms, inventory methods, and record forms that facilitate organizational coordination. The nurse-manager's major responsibility in carrying out these plans is to ensure that they are used correctly and are effective so that staff members have adequate and appropriate materials and use them economically.

Finally, managers are expected to consider existing policies, procedures, and rules when devising new ones specific to the patient-care unit. The fact that all activities that take place in a health-care agency are related to achieving organizational goals cannot be over-emphasized. Because of the interrelatedness of departments, the planning of one usually affects the functions of another. Managerial planning is continuous and is most effective if it is shared with all who are involved in activities being planned.

Nursing Staff Participation in Developmental Planning

Human potential for planning is often not exploited to its fullest in nursing because the nurse tends to concentrate on the individual patient. The attention of the nurse focuses on the nurse-patient relationship; the combination of all the patient's needs at any given time determines the day-to-day goals for management. The pressures of meeting patients' needs on a day-to-day basis often takes precedence in the manager's attention. Continuous problems encountered in giving care or spontaneous thoughts about ways to improve services are often put aside by busy managers. It is necessary to spend some time meditating or reflecting on the services being given on a day-to-day basis to improve the way that services are provided, or to improve the services. Developmental planning is the term used to describe the manager's role in change implementation which begins with thoughtful evaluation of day-to-day activities.

Developmental plans can be short-range or long-range plans that encompass many different aspects of care for all patients served by the health-care agency. In a sense, developmental planning is necessary for adaptation of the organization's functions to the ever-changing needs of patients in a society that is evolving continually. Long-range planning is not only a necessary component of organizational management, but it is also a necessary component of professionalism in nursing. The profession evolves and changes through the activities of nurses who are visionary and who spend time in future planning.

IMMEDIATE VERSUS LONG-RANGE PLANNING

Have you worked on a unit on Tuesday, thinking that everything seemed organized, only to return on Wednesday to find that things were hectic? The expediency of patient care can be identified as a major cause for fluctuating goals for management on the patient-care unit. Patient care is expedient because patient needs cannot be predicted in advance. A hospitalized patient may suddenly develop complications, and a newly admitted patient may have any number or variety of symptoms and needs that must be assessed immediately.

An immediate patient need requires an immediate solution if care is to be beneficial for the patient. Therefore, nurses focus their attention on patient care, which places demands on both their physical and emotional energies. Because of the expediency of care, the present seems more important than future planning.

Managers in nursing are therefore faced with what often seems to be a conflict—planning for the future while meeting the demands of the present. How does one overcome this conflict?

Planning for the future depends on a state of mind, one of thinking in the future while functioning in the present. Two things help the manager to achieve this state of mind. The first is a vision of activities and processes that would improve patient care—a mental picture of what future patient care ought to be. The second is a perspective of the health-care agency's functions, goals, and plans for the future.

The manager should develop a perspective of events that are taking place in the organization. Most organizations have long-range plans for improvement of patient services, such as building construction, expansion of services, or development of new services. Understanding the direction of these plans helps the nurse appreciate the need for planning nursing care in accordance with future plans for the total organization.

The perspective of organizational planning is enhanced if one is aware of the complexity of activities performed within the organization. The following analogy gives a clearer view of the nature of organizational planning.

Imagine that you are in a plane, flying at an altitude of 10,000 feet. The day is clear, and you can see the terrain below. You can see a winding river that forms semicircles that double back on one another. The surrounding earth appears irregular, with crevices, randomly placed trees, and numerous colors breaking the smoothness of its surface. As you continue to watch, a narrow ribbon of pavement draws your attention to a city you are approaching.

In contrast to the random placement of the water, trees, and earth you have just seen, the city appears precise and orderly. Houses are neatly arranged in rows bordered by streets. Water is contained in geometrically shaped pools. You can see tiny automobiles moving evenly along a pattern of streets. It is evident that the city structure has been planned. People have changed the rambling countryside into a configuration that accommodates human activity. The change was brought about because the people were able to think, to make decisions, and to perform activities outlined in their plans to create the city.

The aerial view of the configuration of the city can be compared to the organizational chart pictured in the first chapter. The streets are routes of transportation and provide access to buildings, while the lines of the chart are access lines for authority and for communication. Both configurations represent structural plans that channel human activity, and both facilitate definition of how people formally relate to one another and to their environment. Both the city and the organization have policies, procedures, and rules that govern and direct human activity. However, one has to live in the city or work in the organization to know what actually takes place. One has to be personally involved to fully understand the behavior of people. A cursory view of a city's structure and governing plans only gives an indication of behavior. Similarly, behavior in an organization is only partially determined by the structure and the governing plans.

DRAWBACKS OF SHORT-RANGE PLANNING

Although the city may seem very orderly from the airplane, the configuration may actually be a product of random development over a long period of time. The residents of some cities bemoan the lack of planning and control of the city's growth. Other cities may have benefited from the vision of people who developed plans for the city's growth so that the construction completed in each era would complement that of the others.

Nursing management focusing on the patient's immediate needs is similar to the haphazardly planned city. A decision that meets one patient's needs today may hinder another patient's progress in the future. However, when nursing management is focused on the future, more consideration is given to the implications the decision has for many patients. When this occurs, nursing management is more like that used for developing the planned city.

PLANNING WITHIN LARGER STRUCTURE

Planning in an organization is complex because of the diverse activities that take place in segments of the organization. Consider the diverse activities taking place in the city: The city council is planning for improvement of streets and highways, the school board is planning for transportation of children to and from school, and a church group is debating about where to build the new church. A storekeeper is taking inventory in preparation for a sale, and a family is deciding where to buy shoes for the children.

Organizational activities are also diverse, and this results in separate planning by each department toward accomplishing its own purposes. However, all activities are influenced by the structure and by the governing plans. The family must observe traffic signals when driving to the store to buy shoes. The storekeeper will only open his shop during hours approved by the city council. The school board will have to work within the limits of money available to it.

In the health-care agency people in each department must observe the general rules. Budgets and signals in the organization define boundaries for performance of activities. The nurse who develops a perspective of the total hospital organization realizes how activities of the departments are interrelated. This perspective is the framework in which the nurse operates to apply the management process to achievement of long-range goals that complement those of the total organization.

PROJECTION INTO THE FUTURE

In order to maintain the effectiveness of nursing practice, managers must develop goals which extend beyond the present. These goals may extend over a period of months or years if the management process is to be effectively goal-oriented. This requires projecting into the future.

Through making predictions about changes or trends in giving patient care, managers who are future-oriented identify where they are and then define where they would like to be. The question "How do you think care ought to be given in the future?" will help managers decide what the long-range goals should be.

PROGRESSIVE PLANNING

A manager may find that long-range goals are vague and overwhelming. To overcome these feelings, the manager can institute a method of progressive planning. This method involves analyzing the long-range goal to determine a sequence of subgoals that lead to its achievement. All the subgoals then become short-range goals. By reducing long-range goals to a sequence of realistic and attainable short-range goals, the manager can progress with more assurance of success.

Short-range goals can be used to channel the staff toward effort beyond routine performance of daily work and eventually to achievement of long-range goals they would have considered vague, visionary, and unrealistic. Consistent accomplishment of goals also provides for motivation for staff members to continue the effort to achieve.

An example of a long-range goal you are familiar with is the goal to become a nurse. The sequential development of courses in the school's curriculum gave you realistic short-range goals to accomplish. You achieved a goal each time you passed one of the courses. Your short-range planning was limited to the requirements of each course. Yet, all the while, the broad goal, to become a nurse, gave you direction in your study.

Staff members are similar to students in the way they view goals. Although freshmen student nurses know they want to become graduate nurses, graduation is often a distant, somewhat vague goal. Junior students usually feel more confident than freshmen or sophomores about goal achievement because of their demonstrated ability to accomplish goals. Seniors find that the goal that seemed to be a vision during the freshman year is real and quite near. The curriculum in a school of nursing is planned progressively. The progression of plans provides for consistent and steady direction. It also provides for necessary feelings of accomplishment realized only when goals have been achieved.

FACTORS IN PATIENT CARE

The concept of developmental planning in progressive stages can be applied in nursing management. Planning for long-term goals in nursing begins with determination of measurable factors that remain constant in patient-care situations. These constant factors are those that affect most patients' care. Factors present in almost every patient-care situation can be identified as the patients' common needs, the nursing staff, the patient-care unit, the method for delivering care on the unit, and the health services available in the agency and community. All of these factors are necessary to patient care and all are within the management realm of the nurse.

It is useful to analyze the dimensions of each of these factors separately even though events in one affect the other within the organization. The analysis of events that take place in relation to each factor can be initiated with a brainstorming session. You might ask the question, "How do you think care ought to be given in the future?" Record your answers to this question and then consider what changes would have to be made in each factor or category that is present in most patient-care situations. This is a beginning step in determining the type of data needed to analyze rationally the direction that your change implementation should take. Let us now consider some attributes of each of the factors mentioned to explicate the process of analysis.

Patient Needs. Analysis of patient needs on a given patient-care unit forms the basis for developing long-range plans that will improve care. These plans should be general enough to meet the needs of a number of patients, but specific enough to be applicable to individual patients. General needs can be identified by determining what needs patients tend to have in common. For example, if patients are grouped according to classification of illness on a particular unit, the common needs of patients will in turn be specific to this classification. The nurse is able to develop plans to meet common needs with much greater specificity in a unit largely populated by patients with respiratory diseases than in a unit where patients have a wide range of diseases.

Long-range plans focusing on better methods to meet patient needs include devising more effective ways of caring for the patient's physical and emotional needs, initiating programs that facilitate the patient's rehabilitation, and developing projects for improved patient teaching. The planner asks, "What needs are not being met effectively, and what can be done to improve service to patients?"

The Nursing Staff. Changes for improving the competencies of nursing staff members are based on analysis of each person's ability to give patient care (referred to as a needs assessment). Long-range planning can include development of educational programs to increase nursing knowledge and skill or programs that involve staff members in the development of plans. Staff members who are involved in goal-oriented activities for improving care often learn to improve their personal competency in giving patient care. Analysis of the competencies of staff members enables the planner to identify priorities. Development of staff competencies, for example, should precede their involvement in projects that require advanced knowledge and skill.

The Patient-Care Unit. The process of giving patient care includes performing routine operations that are influenced by both the physical environment of the unit and the organizational policies, procedures, and rules of the total organization. Changes that might improve care can include improved arrangement of equipment and supplies, use of utility rooms, or other alterations in the physical environment that will increase efficiency and effectiveness. Changes can also be made in the organizational structure, policies, procedures, and rules of the unit, in the methods of supplying the unit with the resources it needs to give patient care, and in the methods of communication and cooperation among departments. Analysis of the use of resources and the effectiveness of communication and cooperation is the basis for planning for improvement.

The organization of the patient-care unit and the manager's pattern of leadership influence how long-range plans are developed. In a hospital, for example, the head nurse may be the person who guides all planning for managers on a given patient-care unit. The planner communicates with the head nurse throughout every phase of planning to ensure that efforts to change policy, procedure, or structure will be appropriate for the unit. It is essential that planning by a group of staff members on the unit complements the head nurse's plans for the total unit. Communication between the planner and other medical personnel in relation to plans should be discussed with the head nurse. Sometimes the head nurse gives approval for contacts; at other times the head nurse will represent the staff in contacting other personnel. It is the head nurse's prerogative to set limits for activities conducted on the patient-care unit. The head nurse provides support and guidance in planning and assistance in developing a realistic perspective of the hospital's goals and plans as they relate to the unit.

The Method for Delivering Care. Delivery of health care encompasses methods for providing patient services by the nursing staff as well as that given by personnel in other departments. Patient care can be improved by making changes that are either internal or external to the patient-care unit.

The method used to organize nursing staff is internal and can be analyzed to determine its effectiveness. Does it actually establish effective working relationships among staff members? Does the method support staff members and guide them in giving care? Is the method realistic for staff members' abilities?

Factors external to the patient-care unit include delivery of services by other medical personnel; therefore, analysis of the effectiveness of cooperation among all personnel is a concern for planning. Nurses who work in a hospital, for example, care for patients before and after

they receive health care in other departments. The nurse is the one
health professional who is in constant contact with the hospitalized
patient. Analysis of the effectiveness of interdepartmental cooperation may include questions about the adequacy of patient-care information, expectations of other departments, effectiveness of communication among health professionals for follow-up care, and efficiency in transporting patients to and from departments. The
nurse-manager should play a prominent role in planning efforts
which involve the policies, procedures, and rules established by all
medical personnel.

Resources in the Hospital and the Community. The broad spectrum of
patient needs requires that the nurse in the hospital be concerned
with health services provided both for hospitalized patients and for
people in the community. Patients return to the community when
they are discharged from the hospital. Therefore, the focus of analysis of utilization should be, Do the patients receive "inclusive" care?

There are great variances in services available in communities. Do
members of the nursing staff know about and use health services
available for individual patient care? Is there communication between each service and the hospital? Are there adequate referral
systems for patient utilization of services? Is there sharing of information about patients for continuity of care? These are but a few of
the questions that can be asked in efforts to plan for improved
patient care through utilization of available resources.

It is important that priorities for achieving long-range goals be
established in a realistic way so that the staff members can accept
their participation in the activities. A sequence of short-range goals
should gradually lead staff members to finishing projects while also
increasing their ability to participate in achieving long-range goals.
The long-range goal should continually provide direction and motivation but should not become overwhelming or frustrating for staff
members.

Progressive planning is a stimulus to accomplishment and is a
necessary counterpart of change. The nurse who integrates a futuristic
vision of nursing care with a perspective of the organization's goals
into sound plans for changing the constant dimensions of the
patient-care situation is able to direct the present situation toward the
futuristic vision of patient care. This progressive planning is developmental and supports the long-term growth and stability of the
organization.

Summary

A manager is a key person in an organization. Management is a function of life known to every individual: People organize, activate, control, and evaluate the activities of their lives. Sometimes people carry out these "management processes" without giving thought to the nature of the processes they are using. People who are managers, however, must consciously think about how they use management processes. One can learn to be increasingly efficient and productive as a manager by studying and practicing skills and techniques designed to improve management abilities.

The type of organization, the characteristics of the manager, and the relationship between the manager and the organization all influence how a manager conducts the processes of management. Integration of functions of managers throughout the organization takes place through existing integrating plans such as policies, procedures, and rules. These integrating plans serve also to coordinate the work of the personnel in the entire organization.

Developmental planning is a necessary function of managers and serves to ensure that the integrating plans are evaluated continually and changed in accordance with internal and external changes taking place. Developmental planning is a professional approach to influencing continually the nature of nursing functions and the way that nurses work within organizations. This developmental planning takes place in the social system of the organization and involves all aspects of the organization.

Study Questions

1. Every plan can be divided into three components: a concept of what is to be accomplished, procedures for carrying out the plan, and critical tasks that must be carried out at specific points during activity. Select a plan used for providing care in a health-care agency you are familiar with. Describe this plan according to the three components outlined above.
2. Choose one patient you have cared for and identify the policies, procedures, and rules you used when caring for the patient.
   a. Which of these policies, procedures, and rules are specific to nursing?
   b. Which of the policies, procedures, and rules are general to the total organization?
   c. What methods are used to communicate these policies, procedures, and rules in the health-care agency?
   d. Do the nurses participate in formulating policies, procedures, and rules?

Study Projects

Mary is a group leader on a surgical patient-care unit with a bed capacity of 68. Mary is responsible for the care of 35 patients. Her group comprises three registered nurses and two licensed practical nurses. Her first impression of the unit is that the staff does not communicate well, especially in teaching patients.

Mary realizes that as manager she must integrate her knowledge about the hospital organization, the nursing service organization, the management process, and her vision of staff-patient relationships into a composite of group activities that will improve patient care.

She believes that the primary force for controlling the quality of patient care will be the motivation of each staff member to perform well. Mary's philosophy is that staff members must reach a state of equilibrium in which their motivation is equal to the demands of the work. In keeping with this philosophy Mary makes an initial decision: Improved patient care should be achieved through group process.

Mary then decides to analyze the long-range goals she has for the staff members and for improving patient care. A summary of her analysis reveals the following:

1. The Patients
   a. The majority of patients present problems and needs associated with cardiac diseases.
   b. Patients receive excellent physical care but receive little or no information about the nature of and care required by their condition.
2. The Nursing Staff
   a. RN #1 rotates between days and evenings, relieving the evening nurse two days a week. She has exceptional qualities for assessing patient needs and formulates good care plans that usually are not actualized. She often states that rotating shifts decreases her ability to follow through with the plans. Her ideas are sound and she has a gift for logical thinking, but she must be prodded to share her ideas in a group.
   b. RN #2 has been employed as a part-time nurse for seven years and began full-time employment just three months ago. She is perceptive, efficient, and concentrates on immediate patient needs. She states that her long-term employment as a part-time nurse has caused her to form habits of coming to work, getting the work done, and then going home, forgetting the problems of the day. She then starts the new day free of yesterday's concerns.
   c. RN #3 loves to talk and is well versed in a variety of subjects. She is lively and energetic and is known for her ability to cheer patients. Her favorite subject is cooking so that almost every conference about the patients includes her description of their diets at home.
   d. LPN #1 is a resourceful person who does extra things for patients. She prides herself on her compassion and understanding of patients' reactions to their hospitalization. When care plans are discussed,

she emphasizes emotional aspects of care and never asks a patient to do anything he does not want to do.

   e. LPN #2 is working to make enough money to enroll in a collegiate nursing program. She is curious about pathology and frequently asks about modes of treatment and medications. In conferences she often relates theories from a genetics course she is taking in evening school.

3. Method of Delivering Care

   a. Although the nursing staff is organized in a pattern of group care, the pattern is not totally accepted. It was initiated by the nursing supervisor, who felt that the staff reacted negatively to team method.

   b. The head nurse is well organized and tends to be somewhat authoritarian. She functions well with the unit administrator so that staff needs for materials are adequately met. Usually the head nurse prefers to communicate with staff members individually. She likes to keep records and has copious amounts of data about average length of patient hospitalization, about the most commonly used medications, and about the types and descriptions of emergency situations that occur on the unit.

4. The Patient-Care Unit

   a. Patients' rooms are two-bed rooms with the exception of four private rooms.

   b. The unit administrator is efficient and keeps supplies and communication flowing smoothly among departments. She handles patient needs for administrative services very well.

5. Resources in the Hospital

   a. There is a seven-bed coronary care unit in the hospital. Patients are usually transferred to various patient-care units by the coronary care staff once their condition has stabilized.

   b. The outpatient department has weekly cardiac clinics and material from the Heart Association that is available to patients free of cost.

   c. The laboratory has developed a system for participation in emergency cardiac care and also has several staff members who participate in research.

   d. The hospital has a social service department and qualified dietitians, occupational therapists, and physical therapists.

6. Resources in the Community

   a. There is a well-established Visiting Nurse Association. The nurses care for many chronically ill patients in the community, conduct classes for prenatal care and for bowel and bladder training, and participate in workshops for care of patients with cancer or with special disabling diseases such as multiple sclerosis and cerebral vascular accidents.

   b. A branch office for the American Heart Association is located in the community.

   c. A special civic committee has been formed voluntarily to determine the need for new community services for special groups. Its focus is on the aged, on children with learning disabilities, and on the adolescent.

Mary decides to centralize all the problems in her given situation in the formation of a single long-range goal: *to institute a program for patient teaching.* She has determined the following goals:

1. For the Staff
   a. To unite staff members through use of group process.
   b. To increase each staff member's ability to assess the total needs of patients.
   c. To increase staff members' nursing knowledge about care of patients with cardiac diseases.
2. For the Patient
   a. To minimize the negative effects of the patient's transition from the coronary care unit to the patient-care unit.
   b. To organize a system for providing patients with information and explanations they need about their diseases on a continuous basis, for hospitalization and for after discharge.
   c. To initiate cooperation among all medical personnel who participate in the cardiac patient's care.
   d. To develop a method for evaluating the effectiveness of patient teaching.

Before beginning to work with the staff Mary has determined that:

1. The long-range goal is within the staff's realm of responsibility and ability and that it is approved by the head nurse.
2. The goal is important for improving care and it provides direction for planning.
3. The goal is realistic for the patient-care unit and compatible with the goals of the entire hospital.

Study Questions
1. Evaluate the procedure that Mary has followed to determine her long-range goals. Do you agree with her analysis of the problem?
2. Define short-range goals that will lead to achieving the long-range goal you have determined for this situation.
3. If you were Mary, how would you proceed to incorporate the long-range plans in the performance of management processes?
4. Define the expected functions for Mary as leader of the group and for the staff members as group participants in relation to short-range goals you would plan for:
   a. The organizing phase
   b. The activating phase
   c. The controlling phase
   d. The evaluating phase
5. What impediments do you foresee in achieving the long-range goal Mary has identified?

6. What materials or resources would be helpful to Mary in working with the group?
7. Determine how Mary should communicate the results of the group's activities to others in the organization. What information must be communicated? Who needs the information? What channels and what format should be followed in communicating the information?

References

1. Bernard, C. *The Functions of the Executive* (30th Anniversary ed.). Cambridge: Harvard University Press, 1968.
2. Getzels, J. W., and Guba, E. G. Role, role conflict and effectiveness: An empirical study. *Am. Sociol. Rev.* 19:164, 1954.
3. Shostrom, E. L., and Knapp, L. *Actualizing Therapy: Foundations for a Scientific Ethic.* San Diego: EDITS, 1976.

Suggested Reading

Armstrong, D. M. Nursing administrator's expectations of OR leader. *A.O.R.N.* 25:859–864, April 1977.

Damos, V. R. Management skill: Objectivity. *A.O.R.N.* 25:195–196, Feb. 1977.

Donnelly, J. F. Participative management at work. *Harvard Bus. Rev.* 55:117–127, Jan./Feb. 1977.

Frazier, L. M. Preventive management for supervisors. *Hosp. Top.* 54:21–29, Nov./Dec. 1976.

Godfrey, M. A., and *Nursing '75.* Working conditions. How do yours compare with other nurses? *Nursing '75* 5:85, May 1975.

Hefferin, E. A., and Hunter, R. E. How we turned an idea into a program. Reality orientation. *Nursing '77* 7:88-91, May 1977.

Letellier, M. You can change nursing practice. *Nursing '77* 7:65–66, March 1977.

Lindeman, C. A., and Krueger, J. C. Increasing the quality, quantity, and use of nursing research. *Nurs. Outlook* 25:450–454, July 1977.

Longest, B. B. *Management Practices for the Health Professional.* Reston, Va.: Prentice-Hall, 1976.

McCool, B., and Brown, M. *The Management Response: Conceptual, Technical, and Human Skills of Health Administration.* Philadelphia: Saunders, 1977.

McKain, R. J. *Realize Your Potential.* New York: American Management Association, 1975.

Robinson, V. M. How to initiate change in practice. *A.O.R.N.* 26:54–61, July 1977.

Springate, D. D., and McNeil, M. C. Managemet policies in investor owned hospitals. *Health Care Man. Rev.* 2:57–67, Summer 1977.

3. The Organization of Nursing for Management of Patient Care

There are many variations in the ways that nursing departments are structured. In this chapter we will discuss the types of plans used to organize nursing departments in hospitals and the concomitant management roles of nurses. Some of the major differences among nursing department organizations will be discussed. These include the organization of a patient-care unit, the number of management levels in the nursing department, the placement of the department in the total hospital structure, and finally the patterns of care used to organize nursing staff.

The patient-care unit is the locus of nursing process in the hospital or health-care agency. Since the nursing department exists to support and facilitate the functions of the patient-care units we will first discuss some characteristics of the patient-care unit.

A patient-care unit may be autonomous in its function, its philosophy, and its objectives, but it is also an integral part of the total hospital organization. Personnel from many other departments who provide direct patient-care services and indirect supporting services, such as housekeeping, enter and leave the patient-care unit. These services are important for patient care and therefore must be considered when organizing the structure for patient care on any given unit. The staff nurse who is a manager of care on a patient-care unit needs to be familiar with the organizational plan for the patient-care unit and its relationship to the rest of the hospital. The nurse should also know about the types of medical and supporting services provided by the hospital. Knowledge of the contributions of other professionals helps the nurse plan for efficient and complete patient care. In addition, the nurse should be familiar with the types of services available to patients from the community. The nurse must understand how patients and their families obtain these services in order to provide for continuity of care.

The nurse-manager is concerned with the implications that patients' past and future care have for their current hospitalization. This is particularly important today when hospitals are becoming centers of health-care services. As patients increasingly understand health care, nurses are increasingly involved in helping patients learn about and use health-care services for a wide variety of care measures.

These can include regular physical examinations, particularly if the patient has a chronic health problem, nutritious food, rest, relaxation, immunizations, and care for minor and major acute health problems. The focus of the nurse-manager's functions is patient care, and this focus takes into account the ways the patient learns to use the services of health care.

The Patient-Care Unit

Each patient-care unit has a philosophy and objectives that articulate the scope of the nurse-manager's function. The philosophy and objectives should be written and need periodic review and revision. A philosophy is a broad statement of purpose, while objectives are statements of behaviors to be accomplished by the nursing staff to "activate" the philosophy. The objectives serve as the basis for application of the management processes discussed in Chapter 2: organizing, activating, controlling, and evaluating.

PATIENT-CARE UNIT PHILOSOPHY

You might ask, "Why spend time writing a vague philosophy that no one ever reads again?" It is true that a philosophy may seem general, vague, or more implicit than explicit. It is also true that in articulating a philosophy a group of people must brainstorm. They must explore their ideas in broad perspective, and they must make basic decisions about a definition of nursing care that will serve as a unifying device. When writing a philosophy, members of a group define what they mean by terms such as patient care or rehabilitation. Clarification of ideas, opinions, meanings of terms, and purposes is a necessary part of organizing. A carefully articulated philosophy serves as a common base or focal point for all the ensuing elements of the management process.

The a priori consideration for developing a patient-care unit's philosophy is the patient. Current emphasis on health care as a rapidly growing business has created a recipient of health services who is a consumer rather than an object of health care. Informed consumers ask relevant questions about the services they receive. Managers also should ask themselves questions such as: What is nursing care? Why do patients choose to come to this particular hospital? What do patients expect from the nursing staff? What is the patient's concept of nursing care? What constitutes a successful hospitalization for a patient?

The philosophy should include the nursing staff's description of beliefs about nursing care. Once written, the philosophy should be referred to in subsequent staff activities on the patient-care unit as a reminder of the focus of the staff's efforts. It is interesting to note that because a philosophy is a broad general definition about beliefs of nursing care, it usually remains valid even though the meanings of the words change as nursing-care knowledge evolves. The philosophy must be reviewed frequently, however, to ensure that current interpretation is relevant to current practice.

Unit Objectives. Definition of methods to be used to achieve the purposes stated in the philosophy is the process of formulating specific objectives for patient care. Objectives are clearly stated ways for activating the beliefs in the general statement of philosophy. If the philosophy states that "complete nursing care consists of provision of comfort, teaching patients about care and cure processes, giving support to the patient and family, and planning for the patient's future care needs," the objectives should specifically delineate the behavioral standards expected of the staff for making patients comfortable, for teaching, for giving support, and for health-care planning.

The form used to write objectives is of lesser consequence than is the nursing staff's understanding and acceptance of the objectives. Objectives should be perceived as reasonable and attainable goals by staff. Defining objectives that can be understood and accepted by the entire nursing staff serves to unify the staff members, who then share a common concept of their expectations for giving patient care. An individual nurse, after reading the objectives, should be secure in knowing what is expected, since objectives delineate behaviors required in the care of patients. As you write these behavioral objectives you are actually making decisions about what must be done to achieve the goals stated in the philosophy. Behavioral objectives help the staff know what they are supposed to accomplish. Applying behavioral objectives in giving patient care involves consideration of the physical environment of the unit, the competencies of the staff, and the work to be accomplished. In order to apply objectives more easily it is helpful to categorize them according to similar activities. Objectives so categorized will make it apparent that some activities can be performed in a sequence and some activities are prerequisites for others. Most nursing activities require judgment by the nursing staff to assess the individual patient's needs in terms of the objective. Objectives help the staff organize patient care in a way that facilitates productivity.

The physical environment of the patient-care unit influences how work is organized. For example, an open ward of 20 patients facilitates direct contact of a nurse with several patients at a time; this is not possible when patients are in private rooms. Operational requisites for obtaining supplies and equipment and for activities such as preparing medications, charting, and conferring must be practical for the staff assignments. The physical facility affects how people work together because it influences the way people organize their work and the amount of time it takes to perform an activity. As a manager you must plan to use its good points and devise means to overcome its bad points.

Competencies of the nursing staff will determine how the work ought to be assigned to best meet the objectives. In addition to the staff's competencies, the manager must be aware of hospital and unit policies, job descriptions of staff members, and the unwritten but important relationships that exist among the staff members. With this information the manager can devise objectives that include methods and standards for the work so that the staff members are challenged to use their potential for professional growth in their positions. Writing a philosophy and objectives is part of the organizing process.

Actualizing Objectives. In the activating phase—the time in which staff members perform the work according to the prescribed plan—the manager guides and supports staff functions. Knowledge of how you can best assist staff members in their work is increased if you think of your own experiences as a staff member. What kinds of problems do you have when giving patient care? What type of information was necessary for you? How could you have been helped to provide better care? Information about the staff's collective competencies and about the problems that arise as work is being performed is essential to the manager's participation in the activating element.

Controlling Performance. The objectives of the unit are basic to controlling performance. In order to control the quality of care being given, the manager must control the work and the environment. For example, you may need to assist staff members by obtaining additional supplies, such as linen, so that they may complete the work. You may need to support a staff member who is having difficulty relating to a patient. Another staff member may need assistance to learn how to turn a patient correctly. You may need to confer with a physical therapist about how to coordinate care so that a staff member can organize work better. In control, the manager must reward positive behavior and correct negative behavior. Controlling involves a myriad of activities, all with the purpose of ensuring that care is given in the proper manner and that the work situation provides for smooth functioning of all staff members.

Evaluating Performance. During the time in which the manager is involved in activating and controlling processes, he or she is also involved in evaluating. Because the methods used to give patient care often determine the results, each phase of all activities must be evaluated. Prescribed standards and tools for evaluation are the basis for comparison of what ought to happen with what really happens. Functions of the evaluator include observation, interpreting, recording, and a keen awareness of the interrelationships among events. Continual evaluation is essential for improving patient care and for assisting the staff toward professional growth. Data gathered from evaluation is used to revise or rewrite the unit objectives so that they are updated continually.

All of the care processes and operations of the patient-care unit are supported and facilitated by the nursing department. The scope of managerial roles of nurses in hospitals ranges from the staff nurses on the patient-care units to the director of nursing practice; managerial functions of nurses range from direct patient care to management of the entire nursing department. Intermediate management roles include those of supervisors, or their equivalents, and head nurses. The pattern of organization used in a given nursing department is personified by the management roles.

THE HEAD NURSE

Head nurse is the traditional title for the person who is responsible for managing nursing care on a particular patient-care unit. New titles and positions are being developed in certain instances, but the traditional title is used here. The head nurse usually has a 24-hour responsibility for the patient-care unit, but may be responsible for the unit for a given shift, such as a day head nurse. All activities that take place on the patient-care unit fall into the realm of the head nurse's management. The head nurse sets the tone for relationships among people within the unit. Head nurses have a variable amount of latitude in management of the patient-care unit, but they are usually responsible for developing patterns of patient care, policies, procedures, and rules that are specific to a given patient-care unit, and for following individual prerogatives for giving patient care.

The amount of latitude that the head nurse has in management prerogatives for the patient-care unit depends on the way that the entire nursing department is organized, on the director's interpretation of management roles in the organization, on the types of middle management positions in the nursing department, and on the head nurse's management competencies and perception of his or her own management functions. The head nurse's management style directly affects how staff nurses are expected to function on a given patient-care unit because the head nurse directs all staff and all patient care on the unit.

In addition to the direct patient-care responsibilities, the head nurse participates in providing supporting services to patients. In many instances the head nurse is the liaison person between the patient-care unit and other professionals or other departments. In this regard the head nurse has a coordinating function and establishes networks of communication between the patient-care unit and other departmental personnel. These networks may or may not be formalized in an organizational chart. Head nurses participate in the selection of nursing staff who are employed for the patient-care unit, and in some hospitals they work directly with the personnel department.

THE SUPERVISOR

The supervisory role, like the head nurse role, is a middle management position. The management roles of persons in these intermediate positions are sometimes interchangeable or overlapping. In some hospitals, the head nurse does not report to a supervisor since the head nurse, if knowledgeable, mature, and motivated, needs a minimum of direction. In these hospitals, head nurses often form a peer group for purposes of problem-solving and planning to develop improved methods for giving patient care and to have a source of support.

If there are supervisory positions in the hospital, the supervisor is usually in a pivotal position between the head nurses of several patient-care units and the director of nursing practice or that person's assistant. The supervisor is responsible for management of patient care on a given number of patient-care units, and this person may be more or less directly involved in the processes of giving care. This variance results from different interpretations of the supervisory role among both individual supervisors and different hospitals.

In some hospitals, supervisors manage the operational and mechanical details of the patient-care units, such as arranging for patient services from dietary, laboratory, or x-ray departments. In other hospitals, the supervisor may be a consultant in matters of patient care and is responsible for staff development of head nurses and staff nurses. In yet other hospitals, the supervisor may be a clinical specialist who coordinates the clinical components of patient care. As mentioned previously, the traditional supervisory position may not be found in certain hospitals. When these supervisory positions have been deleted, lay managers or unit administrators are usually employed to take care of management of the operational aspects of the patient-care unit.

THE DIRECTOR OF NURSING

The director of nursing is responsible for the entire nursing department. This person may have an associate or an assistant who performs some aspects of management functions for the department. The scope of the director's managerial role includes definition of the philosophy of the department, formulation of policies that guide all patient-care activities for nursing, establishing working relationships among nurses within the department and between the nursing department and other hospital departments, and ensuring that the department is staffed and that patient care is given within the economic and quality standards of the department. The director interfaces with other management personnel in administrative positions and with community representatives who are involved in hospital functions. Through these contacts, the director interprets nursing to the rest of the hospital personnel at the level of hospital policymaking.

The placement of the department of nursing in the total hospital structure varies. In some hospitals the director has the title of Vice-President for Nursing, a title that implies that the director has a role and responsibility in the central core of the hospital's administrative functions. In other hospitals, the director may be appointed Department Head and may report directly to an administrator of the hospital. Some directors have the title of Clinical Chairman of the Department of Nursing; this title implies that the organization views nursing as a clinical entity on par with other clinical departments such as surgery or medicine. Placement of the department and of the director's role influences not only how nursing is perceived by others in the organization, but also the scope of nursing functions in the organization.

As discussed in Chapter 1, the type of organizational structure influences the management roles of personnel. In a tall, traditional bureaucratic structure, the locus of control for decisions made in the department of nursing tends to be at the level of the director. In flat, decentralized structures, the control is disseminated throughout the nursing department. The responsibility for decision-making tends to follow the lines set forth in the organizational structure, but it can be delegated or not according to the director's philosophy and management style.

The director's philosophy of nursing is demonstrated in several ways. How the director defines the expectations of nurses, determines the criteria for effectiveness of patient care and for nursing staff performance evaluations, clarifies nursing functions, and initiates projects for nursing development, all reflect the director's philosophy. The director interprets nursing roles not only to nurses but also to other hospital personnel. Since the director is accountable for all patient care given by nurses, the director's beliefs will determine what he or she considers important in implementing plans that ensure accountability.

One of the director's functions is to determine the boundaries for nursing practice in the hospital, which in turn establishes the working relationships of nurses in the hospital. The structure or pattern of interaction that the director establishes reflects his or her concepts about nursing and management style. In practice, most directors use different management styles according to the requirements of a particular situation. The director's use of management styles affects the way that all nurses in the department adapt to different situations, since there is a tendency for people to manage as they are managed. The three major types of management styles discussed in the traditional literature include authoritarian, democratic, and laissez-faire.

AUTHORITARIAN MANAGEMENT

An authoritarian management style implies that the manager makes all of the decisions or maintains control over decision-making. The authoritarian manager often expects each person to comply with policies, procedures, and rules and tends to employ people who respond well to structure and who will comply with directives. Some characteristics of an authoritarian manager can be gleaned from the following description of a nursing-department director.

Mrs. Jones believes strongly that if she is to be responsible for the nursing department, she must make the major decisions that relate to nursing. She holds weekly meetings with the head nurses and informs them of plans and activities she expects them to conduct on their units. Every other day, Mrs. Jones meets with the supervisors to discuss problems. Following these meetings she decides which problems require action and makes decisions accordingly. These decisions are usually announced at the following meeting. She handles problems efficiently and is able to give clear and concise directions. When you talk to her you feel that she really listens, but you know she is sorting out your comments and will do something only about the problems she thinks are important.

DEMOCRATIC MANAGEMENT

The democratic management style implies that decision-making extends throughout the organization. The democratic style involves others in identification of problems, in analysis of alternative courses of action, and in making decisions. The democratic manager communicates openly with the staff to ensure that decisions are in keeping with the organizational and departmental goals.

The democratic manager tends to work with groups in carrying out management functions. Group process is used to involve staff members, to facilitate their growth, to give them the opportunity to control their own activities, and to increase competency through participation. An outcome of working in groups to make decisions is that all group members have a chance to provide input and to work through problems, thereby increasing their understanding of decisions and giving them an opportunity to make a commitment to these decisions.

LAISSEZ-FAIRE MANAGEMENT

The laissez-faire management style is associated with an easygoing approach to management in which staff members have the freedom to make their own decisions. The person who uses the laissez-faire management style gives people latitude to follow their own prerogatives in determining their working relationships and in formulating policies, procedures, and plans. This type of management usually results in a loosely organized department and is beneficial when the manager wishes to stimulate creativity and innovation.

APPLICATION OF DIFFERENT MANAGEMENT STYLES

Managers often shift from one management style to another according to different situations, although the manager may have a predominant style. In order to apply management styles effectively, the manager assesses the staff members' needs for direction and evaluates the situation in which the managerial decisions are being made. Since the director sets the tone for the entire nursing department, the director can be perceived as beginning a chain reaction of relationships among employees through use of management styles. A supervisor or head nurse has similar influence on people they manage, just as a staff nurse influences relationships of others depending on the way that management styles are applied.

An example of the way that different management styles can be applied by the same person is given in the following notation.

Mrs. Green, Director of Nursing, has three major goals in mind for her staff. The first is development of criteria for evaluation of quality patient care. The second concerns formulation of policies for cooperation of hospital nurses with the Visiting Nurse Association in the community. The third is to develop an innovative pattern of organizing the department.

Each week Mrs. Green meets with the supervisors and the head nurses to explore methods for developing criteria for evaluation of care. The group first identified the value of developing the criteria and are now absorbed in establishing a survey of what actually happens on the patient-care unit. Thus far Mrs. Green has not intervened in group decisions, but she often clarifies alternatives in procedures when necessary. She has given the group complete control of definition of their own methods.

For several weeks Mrs. Green has been meeting with representatives of the Visiting Nurse Association to determine how they might establish a cooperative relationship with the hospital for referral of patients. She has worked with the director of the Visiting Nurse Association to develop a set of guidelines that she plans to present to the supervisors at their weekly meeting. At that time she will define the guidelines, explain their rationale, and outline a plan for initiating referral forms on all the units.

For the third goal Mrs. Green has formed a special committee of nursing personnel, representative of all management roles. This committee has been given complete freedom to develop new and different plans for organizing the nursing department. Mrs. Green does not attend the meetings unless invited and has assured the group that their final plan will be presented to the group of supervisors and head nurses when it is completed by the committee.

In the first instance Mrs. Green is using a democratic management style to establish criteria for evaluating the quality of patient care. She chose this style for the specific purpose of obtaining the support of the staff through their involvement and participation in the planning stages. She believes that this involvement is a requisite of effectively conducting a project to evaluate patient care because the staff must understand the criteria if they are to apply them effectively to the work situation.

She has chosen to use the authoritarian management style in establishing a relationship with the Visiting Nurse Association. Factors which led to this decision were the personality of the director of the Visiting Nurse Association and the fact that all details inherent in the decisions were administrative in nature. The director of the Visiting Nurse Association appreciates authority and functions better in a one-to-one situation than in a group when plans are being discussed. In time, both directors plan to involve their staffs in this planning, but both wish to work out the details before presenting a project to their staffs.

Finally, Mrs. Green has chosen to use the laissez-faire method of management for the committee that is developing an innovative plan for establishing methods of care. She has done this because she believes that the staff will be more creative and innovative in a loosely organized structure. She sincerely desires to initiate an innovative plan and believes that the staff members who are directly affected by the pattern of care on the patient-care unit will consider factors she would not have thought of.

THE STAFF NURSE

A staff nurse's functions are concerned with management of a group of patients and sometimes with the management of other staff nurses and nonprofessional personnel. All of the other managerial personnel in the nursing department serve to support and facilitate the staff nurse's function. Staff nurses are crucial in nursing management since patient care is the central purpose of the nursing department, and staff nurses give patient care. The staff nurses' functions are not only supported by managerial personnel in the nursing department, but also by the entire organizational structure of the hospital.

Patterns for organizing nursing staff on a patient-care unit have changed over the years through a process of evolution. The present methods used in hospitals for organizing nursing staff differ and often reflect major characteristics of patterns that have been popular in the past. These patterns are changing continually. Projections for future patterns can be made by evaluating the best features of those used in the past. The following descriptions of major patterns used in hospitals over time indicate how stages of development have occurred to the present time.

Organization of Nursing Services

Historically, patterns of organizing nurses in the United States have paralleled changes in the country's social climate. Each era has influenced the development of change in the next era. The changes have occurred gradually and at different rates in different hospitals. For this reason it is possible to find features representative of each era in present organizational patterns.

SCHOOLS OF NURSING

Organization of nursing services in this country can be traced back to its founding. However, the first major development that continues to affect today's nursing began with the establishment of nursing schools in hospitals in the 1870s. At this time the Victorian era was on the decline, and women were becoming actively involved in providing service to others through organizations. Some of the first schools of nursing in the country were initiated by groups of women who cooperated with others in their communities to improve care for hospitalized patients.

These early schools brought young women into hospitals to learn the practice of nursing. The learning process was a combination of a few classes concerned with the basic elements of patient care and much clinical practice. For the most part, the students learned nursing by providing patient care under the supervision of graduate nurses. The students actually staffed the hospitals, and following graduation they were usually employed by families as "private-duty" nurses. Some nurses remained in hospitals to assume the roles of administrator, executive overseer, and teacher. These people formed the management structure for the nursing department.

Perhaps the greatest contribution to nursing resulting from the establishment of schools of nursing is the fact that students proved the value of having trained nurses provide care in hospitals. By proving their worth for improving patient care, they established a need for nursing in hospitals that has increased throughout the years. Today we assume that nurses are essential for the care of hospitalized patients.

The Case Method

The next era of change in organizing nursing patterns came about as a result of the depression of 1929. Few families could afford a live-in nurse during the depression, and many graduate nurses returned to the hospital to seek employment. From necessity they agreed to work for room and board. The influx of graduate nurses led many hospitals to close their schools because students were no longer needed to staff the hospital.

Nurses at this time were accustomed to using the case method for giving care. Practice in homes reinforced their concept that they should care for the complete needs of the patient. The large numbers of nurses living in the hospital made it possible for them to continue using the same method. This meant that every nurse was responsible for giving complete care to her own patients. Today this method is still used by students in schools of nursing. The student focuses attention on meeting the complete needs of a patient who is usually representative of a particular type of patient needs that the student is studying in class. A recreation of the case method is used increasingly in current practice and is termed primary nursing. It was formerly thought that this method was very expensive in terms of professional nurse salaries, but current data indicate that primary nursing is an economical pattern of care delivery.

The case method remained the most prevalent pattern for giving care in the hospital until World War II. In the interim, medical care gradually increased in complexity. The growth of private and public health insurance plans in conjunction with development of medical technology led to increasing numbers of patients entering hospitals for treatment. Increased use of hospitals ensured the continuing employment of nurses.

During the period prior to World War II the role of nurses expanded. The focus of nursing has always been to provide patient care. Nurses in early schools were concerned with providing comfort and a safe environment for patients. Care consisted of providing a clean environment with proper ventilation, bodily comfort, and nutritious diet. Nurses were responsible for the total scope of such activities as bathing patients, preparing and serving food, and cleaning the patients' rooms.

As medical diagnosis and treatment became more complex, nurses retained their environmental care and comfort functions and took on new functions such as taking blood pressures and body temperatures and assisting in surgical procedures. The increasing sophistication of patient care created a need for medically related areas of practice for provision of special patient services, such as x-ray and laboratory procedures.

Nurses gradually assumed increasing responsibility for coordinating the patient care provided by all medical personnel. This coordination required channeling patients to other departments of the hospital, requisitioning services and equipment, reporting to increasing numbers of personnel, and coping with desk work. The changes in patient care also broadened the supervisor's function of coordination of services, leaving less time for working with staff or direct patient contact.

The Functional Method

World War II provided impetus for the next major change in organizing nursing staff. Many nurses left hospitals to care for soldiers at the battlefront, and hospitals were staffed with volunteers, aides, and graduate nurses who remained at home. The numbers of graduate nurses were increased through plans, such as the Cadet Nursing Program, that enabled many young people to enter nursing.

To ensure better utilization of the large numbers of personnel with different educational preparation then employed to provide patient care, and to cope with the rapid expansion of the nurse's role due to medical developments resulting from the war, the functional pattern of organization was developed. In this method, functions were assigned to staff members in accordance with their preparation and abilities. The professional nurse assumed the functions of communicating with physicians, carding orders, giving direction to subprofessional staff members, administering medications, and giving treatments. Nurse's aides performed more technical care measures, such as taking temperatures and giving baths. Assigning tasks according to ability and education provided for efficiency during the time when professional nurses were scarce.

In the 1940s Licensed Practical Nurses achieved formal recognition so that there were legally two levels of prepared practitioners: the professional nurse and the practical or vocational nurse. Patient needs continued to be categorized in terms of functions of the nursing staff. In addition to being an efficient method, the functional pattern also ensured that personnel performed the tasks for which they were prepared with supervision from professional nurses.

The functional method is still employed in some hospitals, especially in situations in which there is a lack of professional staff. Some hospitals may use a different pattern for staff organization during the day shift, reverting to use of the functional pattern for the evening and night shifts.

One result of the functional pattern of assigning duties has been fragmentation of patient care. It is reasonable to assume that when staff members concentrate on meeting specific and segmented patient needs they become task-oriented. An example of a task-oriented nurse is the "medicine nurse" whose role is administering medications to all the patients day after day. When giving the medications, this nurse focuses on expediently carrying out the task rather than on the complete needs of the patient. When the functional method is used, efforts must be made to stimulate staff to develop a perspective of total patient needs rather than a limited view that relates only to their specific function.

The Team Method

Team nursing emerged as a solution to the problem created by fractioning patient care. The basis for the team pattern is the concept of democracy. Through the team, the talents and skills of nurse's aides, licensed practical nurses, and registered nurses are united in a group. Members of the group share in the care of a number of patients. Participation in group activities gives members an opportunity to develop their abilities to provide patient care.

RESPONSIBILITIES OF THE TEAM LEADER

Organization of staff members in the team pattern places great responsibility on the team leader. The leader must be able to influence members of the team and must be secure in the knowledge of patient care and in the ability to work with groups. The leader is responsible for planning and evaluating the patient care provided by all team members while simultaneously identifying and developing their nursing skills through group activities. Team members depend on the direction and guidance of their leader. It is most important that the leader have a concept of teamwork because this concept is a requisite for the effectiveness of the team pattern for organizing staff.

TEAM ACTIVITIES AS MANAGEMENT TECHNIQUES

The team nursing method includes a series of activites that are conducted with groups of team members. These activities are management techniques that enable the leader to provide for guidance and growth of the team members. They include assignment conferences, patient-centered conferences, and development of nursing-care plans. Each has a specific purpose.

Assignment conferences provide an opportunity to impart information about patient care and can also be used as planning conferences in which staff members make decisions about how they will work together. Patient-centered conferences give staff members an opportunity to express feelings and attitudes, discuss patient needs, and define solutions to patient-care problems. Nursing-care plans provide for continuity of care. They are written statements of goals and objectives for care and summarize nursing measures that are used by all who care for patients. All team members participate in designing nursing-care measures appropriate to specific patient needs.

These management techniques promote communication among staff members and involve them in learning more about patient care through participation in planning and evaluating patient care. The differences in educational preparation and experience among staff members are minimized through group participation. The knowledge and skills of the professional nurses on the team are shared with subprofessionals through cooperation in giving care and through continued exchange of ideas.

These management techniques can become routines when used by a leader who does not incorporate the concept of teamwork in relationships with staff members. If staff members perceive them as nonproductive experiences, conducted only because it is so prescribed, they lose their value.

TEAM NURSING AS AN ATTITUDE

Team nursing is perhaps more an attitude than a method. This attitude is one of "participative democracy" in achieving goals. The following excerpt from a team leader's diary affords insight into the thoughts and feelings of the leader:

7:00 A.M.   Attended report given by the night nurse. We made rounds for the sickest patients, and the night nurse demonstrated use of the new chest suction apparatus for Mr. T.

7:30 A.M.   Updated assignments made yesterday—changed the assignment for Mrs. X., the nurse's aide, because the RN should take care of Mr. T., the new patient with chest tubes . . . I think I really made sure that team member's abilities were matched with patient needs.

8:00 A.M. Conducted assignment conference. The new nurse's aide is getting the idea—she actually told me what she planned to do for Mr. J. today. I was pleased with the depth of her thinking! Also with the way she and the RN spontaneously planned how they would cooperate in caring for their patients—it is true that each needs the other's help. Everybody discussed specific goals for patient care for the day. . . .

Also posed the problem: how can we better care for Mrs. S.? Such a difficult patient! Set time for a conference to discuss her care. Hope all the team members were well informed and stimulated.

Made rounds—observed care given and talked to patients, to doctors, to therapists. Revised nursing-care plans!! Helped NA with Mrs. S. Talked with Mr. J. about his new diet. Helped LPN get Mr. R. up for the first time. Must decide what to do about Mrs. M.—gave her a bath as a way to evaluate her condition more fully and to get to know her.

11:30 A.M. Lunch with the NA—had to find out what she thinks about her responsibilities! She hasn't really participated in a conference yet.

12:00 More patient care—little Mrs. S. is a challenge. Gave advice, clarified-taught-evaluated. Had to change the RN's assignment—admitted a *very* sick patient this afternoon. Helped NA write new ideas on Mrs. S.'s care plan.

2:00 P.M. Had a good discussion about Mrs. S. at patient conference. Will explain the use of the new disposables tomorrow. Have to prepare a conference about continuity of care for next week—also have to dream up a project for the team. Maybe the group should do the dreaming!

2:20 P.M. Mrs. S. again—hoped to get her settled—talked with her son and think he understands her care better now. Made out assignments for tomorrow—got organized for report too. One final check to make sure that everything is O.K.

3:00 P.M. Gave report—P.M. nurse has some good ideas about Mrs. S. Together we will cure her. Our motto is continuity.

3:30 P.M. End of a busy day—the team spirit is improving.

DIFFICULTIES RELATED TO TEAM MANAGEMENT

From this excerpt you can get an idea of the scope of the team leader's activities. Because of the many demands on the team leader's time, some of the management techniques, such as conferences, seem to be extraneous to the immediate needs of patients. When the team leader finds it difficult to conduct group activities, the team method loses some of its meaning for the staff.

Other potential drawbacks of the use of the team method for providing patient care are related to staffing. When the team leader and team members change from day to day, the benefits of team nursing cannot be realized because team members must work together for a period of time if the concept of team nursing is to be useful. Have you heard nurses say, "How can you have a team with only two staff members?" or "The staff turnover rate is so great that the same nurses rarely work together," or "How can I conduct a conference when I'm supposed to admit all of those new patients and then give reports?"

OTHER PATTERNS FOR STAFF ORGANIZATION
The team concept can be applied to almost every pattern of staff organization. Other, similar patterns have been developed on the same basic premise as team nursing—that group interaction is beneficial for giving patient care. Some of these patterns are referred to as group care or cluster care. Like team nursing they organize groups of staff, including nurse's aides, licensed practical or vocational nurses, and registered nurses, for the purpose of providing patient care. The mix of nursing staff can vary in group or cluster care patterns. These patterns are different from team nursing in that the numbers of staff in a group or cluster are fewer and the numbers of patients are also reduced.

Primary Nursing Care
Primary nursing care, initiated at the University of Minnesota Hospitals in Minneapolis, Minnesota, is emerging as an organizational pattern for giving nursing care that meets criteria of quality care and job satisfaction. Primary nursing care is most similar to the case method in that it emphasizes the nurse's involvement in meeting the patient's total care needs. This pattern of care enables the primary nurse to form an in-depth relationship with the patient in providing care that involves the patient in decision-making.

THE PRIMARY NURSE ROLE
The underlying philosophy of primary nursing care is that the primary nurse provides comprehensive care that is continuous throughout the patient's stay in the hospital and during the phase immediately following hospitalization. The primary nurse has a caseload of primary patients and is autonomous in application of clinical nursing knowledge and skill in their care. The primary nurse is accountable for the processes and the outcomes of care for assigned patients. Patients are assigned to primary nurses on the basis of their needs

and the primary nurse's competencies. The primary nurse has 24-hour responsibility for these patients and the related needs of their families and is assisted in their care by associate nurses.

Among the activities included in the primary nurse's role are taking a nursing history on admission and sometimes conducting a physical examination. On the basis of data collected in this assessment and from the physician's plan for medical care, the primary nurse initiates the patient's nursing-care plan. The primary nurse cares directly for the patient during one shift and is assisted in the patient's care during the other two shifts by designated associate nurses. These associate nurses follow the nursing-care plan initiated by the primary nurse and contribute to it as needed. Assignments are consistent so that the same nurses care for the patient during his or her hospitalization. The primary nurse makes decisions about the patient's nursing care and coordinates the patient's care with other hospital personnel who contribute to the care. Primary nurses maintain a colleagueship with physicians in which the medical plan of care and the nursing plan are integrated. The primary nurse is directly responsible and accountable for the patient's care, and directs and coordinates care given by the associates.

ASSIGNMENTS IN PRIMARY NURSING

The types of assignments used for primary nursing vary [11, 12]. In some instances, the primary nurse has five or so primary patients. In other situations, the nurse may have two or three primary patients and may be an associate nurse for two or three other patients. Sometimes only selected patients have primary nurses. When this is the case, the remainder of the patients are cared for in groups by groups of staff, using a modified team or cluster care approach. Modular nursing has been developed in some settings to bridge the gap between team nursing and primary nursing [1, 8, 14].

MODULAR NURSING: A BRIDGE TO PRIMARY NURSING

Modular nursing is a modified form of team nursing in which a registered nurse and either a licensed practical nurse or a nurse's aide form a module to take care of a group of eight to ten patients. The licensed practical nurse or nurse's aide is assigned to the registered nurse, who plans, implements, and evaluates the patients' care and directs, guides, and supervises the care given by the LPN or aide. The ratio of patients for each module varies according to the acuity of the patient's condition and the shift time. Usually the ratio is higher during the night shift.

JOB DESIGN FOR PRIMARY NURSING MODELS

Primary nursing models incorporate principles of effective job design. Because primary nurses are able to follow through with all steps of the nursing process personally in caring for their patients they develop a sense of "ownership" or territory in their patient assignments. This pattern of care presents the nurse with a personal challenge to be competent, to apply knowledge and skill, to grow in clinical expertise, and to be accountable and responsible for the process and outcomes of care. The feedback from evaluation reflects directly on the care that the primary nurse has given.

Research conducted to determine effective job designs for professionals supports the importance of job challenge and accountability. Hall and Lawler's study of professional research and development personnel [5], for example, indicates that these professional workers considered working in-depth on a small number of projects to be more challenging than working on a number of different projects. The challenge and responsibility associated with in-depth involvement in a small number of projects led to high levels of job satisfaction, which in turn served to motivate the professionals to achieve high levels of performance. The results of this study illustrate why nursing staff members respond favorably to the primary nursing model.

Hall and Lawler also found that job pressure could be related to challenge. They define pressure as "experience of a particular force," which is different from conflict. Conflict is defined as "opposition of two or more pressures." The pressures they studied included internal pressure to be competent exerted by the professional and external pressure from the organization to produce quality performance. They considered these to be positive pressures since there was congruence between the internal pressure in the individual and the external pressure from the organization. The pressures these researchers found to be positive included not only satisfying needs but also dealing directly with budgetary control and relating directly with the client.

Hall and Lawler believe that the job design for the professional who has high needs to achieve and to be successfully competent should provide for stretching the employee's capabilities. The job design has to allow the professional to demonstrate competence, to visibly influence the environment, and to grow in professional competence. They postulate that when the professional is successfully competent, his or her needs are satisfied and this satisfaction leads to continued effort. Hackman [4] writes that core job dimensions in job design are variety in skills, identity with the tasks, significance of the tasks, autonomy, and feedback. He has developed a model in which these job dimensions are shown to be related to the employee's "psychological state" in creating job satisfaction. The variety, identification, and significance of the work are related to the meaningfulness of the work for the individual while autonomy is related to the responsibility a person feels for the work. Knowledge of results of one's work or feedback is necessary for continued satisfaction. Primary nursing fulfills the criteria for meaningful work by providing for variety in giving care. When a nurse is assigned a caseload of primary patients this nurse identifies with the care given and believes that this care is significant. The primary nurse has more autonomy than team members, and also receives more direct feedback about the results of the work because of the direct nurse-patient relationship.

Nurses have a reputation for short tenure in staff nurse positions and for high mobility, which is possible because they can be employed in hospitals throughout the country to perform similar nursing-care functions [10]. Although nurses who are employed by hospitals are dependent on the hospital environment for supporting services and for the environment for giving nursing care, they do not necessarily have to have a strong identification with any given hospital to function. Because of the high costs of orientation and of turnover [9], efforts to make staff nursing positions more satisfying to nurses are worthwhile fiscally. If the performance of the staff nurses increases in quality, the organization benefits from their increased productivity and from the increased satisfaction of patients.

Primary nursing care has proved to be an effective job design for increasing staff nurses' satisfaction. It has also been demonstrated that primary nursing care increases patient satisfaction. Daeffler [3] demonstrated that patients perceived that they gained more information about their care, were taught about their care more fully, and experienced fewer omissions in care when the primary nursing care design was used. There are also many reports in the literature that substantiate these findings [1, 8, 12, 14]. In many instances, patients who have experienced primary nursing care have requested their primary nurse on return admissions to the hospital. These patients perceive that primary nursing care provides them with a care-giver who is also a teacher, a counselor, an advocate and a liaison between the patient and other health services and community health-care agencies during hospitalization and following discharge. In some settings, the primary nursing model includes an extended care function for the primary nurse, who makes home visits and who maintains contact with the patient for solving care problems following discharge.

Organizational Implications of Primary Nursing

Primary nursing care has implications for the total hospital organization. To be effective, this model requires that the staff be professional. Some hospitals have phased out employment of nurse's aides when changing to primary nursing care. Marram [12] found that nurses who gave higher quality care were more idealistic and professional. This finding has also been demonstrated in other studies concerned with evaluating the effectiveness of primary nursing care.

CLINICAL NURSING EMPHASIS

Another implication primary nursing care has for the organization is that it focuses nursing activities on clinical nursing. Primary nursing care changes the head nurse's function, and it also changes the role of the head nurse and of staff nurses in procurement of supplies and services. Many authorities cite that it is important that there be a position such as a unit administrator or unit secretary to take over this type of function so that the nurses are free to give patient care. In the primary nursing care model, the primary nurses report to the head nurse, who is responsible for the delivery of all nursing care given on the unit. The head nurse is most effective in the primary care model if he or she is a competent behavioral model for primary nurses. A clinical specialist or a person with clinical expertise [1, 12] appears to be the most effective behavioral model.

PROFESSIONAL GROWTH

Primary care nurses become increasingly involved in developing their own clinical expertise. This motivation to continue learning requires that the head nurse assume a major role in day-to-day staff development and that continuing education programs based on a needs assessment of the nursing staff be provided. Increased involvement with patients and their families or significant others stimulates primary nurses to upgrade clinical knowledge and skills in interviewing, communication, methods for integrating families in patient care, patient teaching, and assessment. These nurses can concentrate on clinical nursing care rather than on spending their time performing tasks or directing and supervising the care given by nonprofessional nursing staff.

COST EFFECTIVENESS

An important consideration in change implementation represented by the development of primary nursing care is the cost effectiveness of the new model. A number of studies have been conducted to compare the costs of primary nursing care with the costs of team nursing or of functional nursing [1, 11, 14]. There is increasing evidence that primary nursing care models do not cost more than the other two models. Even though primary nursing care requires increased numbers of professional nurses, savings can be realized because of many factors. Corpuz [1] cites the inefficient use of time by nurse's aides, whose functions are restricted to specific tasks; the costs of orientation, training, directing, and supervising nurse's aides by professional nurses; the associated overextension of professional nurses, who are responsible for both patient care and for directing and supervising care given by nonprofessionals; and the tendency of nurses to be task-oriented rather than patient-care oriented in the functional and team methods as reasons why primary nursing care is cost-effective.

PROFESSIONAL INNOVATION

Primary nursing care stimulates innovation by professional nurses because these nurses tend to identify with and "live" in the patient's world. As a result, the primary nurses are more aware of the patient's problems and assume an advocacy role in helping the patient to use health-care services effectively and to assume an active role in his or her own care. The primary nurses are not distracted by tasks or functions that are not directly related to their patients' care. The primary nursing care model is a form of decentralized organization in which decision-making is disseminated throughout the organization. For many nurses, changing from a bureaucratic organizational structure in a nursing department to such a decentralized structure is difficult. Techniques of change implementation discussed in Chapter 8 are usually necessary when the change to primary nursing care is made in a hospital. Many of these nurses not only have to change their fundamental role concept of nursing, but they also have to learn many of the human behavior skills that are required by the one-to-one nurse-patient relationship that is the locus of primary nursing care.

EFFECTS OF CHANGE ON THE ORGANIZATION

When changing the pattern of care to a new one such as primary nursing care, it is necessary to involve others in the organization in the change. The administrators of the hospital, for example, often have to adapt to the primary care model by changing methods for supplying the patient-care units and for maintaining the patient-care unit environment. If these changes are to be made and made effectively, administrative personnel should be knowledgeable about the goals, methods, benefits and needs that primary nursing care will initiate.

Primary nursing care can be a stimulus to the development and maintenance of professional attitudes in a nursing department. To be effective, nurses have to accept the responsibility, accountability, and authority implied by primary nursing care. In addition, these nurses have to be supported by the organizational structure. There is a potential for conflict between the professionals and the organization, since innovation is an aspect of professionalization but not of bureaucratization [2, 6]. R. H. Hall [6] states that professionalization can take place within a bureaucratic structure if the structure provides for coordination and communication that facilitates the professional's performance. The potential for conflict between the two arises from differing interests in regard to the professional's goals, application of knowledge, the complexity of professional tasks, and the professional's need to control resources. When the organization allows professionals to perform complex tasks according to their specified body of knowledge and code of ethics, there need not be conflict.

Thus far the primary nursing care model has proved to be effective in many hospitals. As with any pattern of organization or job design, the specific requisites of the primary nurse's role vary among hospitals. It could be speculated that one of the reasons for the effectiveness of primary nursing care is that both nurses and patients are gaining more recognition. Nurses who are changing to the primary nursing care model gain recognition through the "halo" effects of the stimulation of being involved in change (Chap. 8). Patients receive greater recognition through the improved performance of the primary nurses that results from their increased motivation to be competent. These effects are desirable, since they promote innovation and increased quality.

EFFECTIVENESS OF VARIOUS CARE PATTERNS

There is, at this time, no universal "most desirable" pattern for giving nursing care because of the diversity in hospitals and the differences in availability of professional nurses in various regions of the country. All nurses can, however, use the best aspects of all patterns of care to devise a pattern that suits their situation. Primary nursing care, for example, uses some of the management techniques that are also part of team nursing activities, such as nursing-care plans, patient-centered conferences, and measures for continuity of care. Modular nursing also uses some of the concepts of team nursing, such as group interaction. It differs in the span of control for the leader; the modular leader relates to fewer staff and patients and thus concentrates on patient care more than on staff direction. These are two examples of how components of different patterns of care can be recombined to form new patterns.

Many nurses have become accustomed to working in groups through their experiences in team nursing, group nursing, or cluster-care patterns. There are certain advantages that can be gained by employees through group participation in care. Some of these will be discussed in the following chapter. There are also advantages to practicing nursing in an autonomous fashion with associates, such as in primary nursing care. Hackman has written that ". . . as yet there are no simple or generally accepted criteria for a well designed job . . . and it is not clear whether work should be structured to be performed by individuals or by a group of employees working together" [4]. How nurses best work together changes with their role perceptions and with the changing normative expectations of the times. One of the current changes taking place in nursing is the increased educational level for nurses who are becoming clinical specialists. This development, associated with expansion in nurses' roles will probably have a great impact on the future developments of patterns of giving care in hospitals.

Specialized Nursing Care

The expansion of the nurse's role has gained momentum since World War II. Because patient needs have become more definitive through rapid growth of specialized medical knowledge, nursing has become increasingly complex. New developments in organizing patient care in health-care agencies are evolving in relation to specialization in medical care and the rapid growth of medical technology.

Efficient hospital administration involves grouping similar services together in a common geographic location. Services can be categorized in several ways, such as according to phases of illness or types of disease. Progressive patient care categorizes services by phases of illness including intensive care, intermediate care, convalescent care, self-care, and home care. This is an example of arranging hospital services according to the special needs of patients. The establishment of care units for patients with specific phases of illnesses fosters specialization of nursing skills. Categorization of patient needs according to phases also enables nurses to specialize in care for patients with acute or chronic illnesses. Special care units give nurses the option of developing competencies in a given area of practice. Some nurses feel that this specialization generally results in personal involvement, growth, and job satisfaction.

Another way of categorizing patient services is by type or classification of illness. Coronary care, renal dialysis, and neurological care units are typical of special care units. These special units have given impetus to development of the nurse-clinical specialist who becomes knowledgeable about the medical technology and related nursing care in a specialty area. One can become a clinical specialist through experience in giving care on a specialized nursing unit or through advanced study of a clinical specialty in a graduate nursing program.

Job descriptions and interpretations of the roles of clinical specialists reflect variations in the way different nursing departments organize care. In some hospitals the clinical specialist serves as a consultant who guides and directs other nurses in giving patient care. In other hospitals the clinical specialist assumes management responsibilities similar to those of a supervisor. Yet other hospitals employ clinical specialists who concurrently give nursing care and teach students and those who care for patients only during the critical phases of illness or in periods of stress. These nurses' work schedules are often determined by the patients' needs for their expertise.

There are presently no universally accepted roles for the nurse-clinical specialists and no common patterns of care which include such specialists. The nursing profession is evolving in the development of increasing numbers of nurse practitioners functioning independently or in joint practice, in private practice, and in various types of health-care agencies. Future roles for nurses, while a matter of speculation, appear to be advancing toward more autonomous and professional expertise. Hall [7] illustrates this change in description of new definitions of nursing practice in state statutes that regulate the practice of nursing.

Only recently have nurses begun to rid themselves of tasks inherent in the management of physical and material aspects on the patient-care unit. Ward secretaries are now trained to assist nurses by performing such tasks as transcribing orders, answering the phone, and relaying messages. Unit managers have been employed by many hospitals to take care of such management aspects of the unit as obtaining equipment and supplies and coordinating the functions of units with the total hospital operation. When these services are available, nurses are able to consider their roles in terms of managing direct patient care.

Nurses participate in activities for developing the changing health-care system in daily nursing practice. This participation requires that all medical personnel coordinate their efforts to prevent segmentation of care and to provide for continuous care. Nurses can become "change agents" in patient care and must control their own practice of nursing. This control must foster progressive change in patterns used to manage patient care.

Study Questions

1. A student gradually formulates a concept of the nurse's role when studying nursing. This concept is influenced by the instructor's expectations of students as well as by the behaviors of nurses who are practicing in the health-care agencies that employ nurses.
   a. Consider your own concept of nursing. How were you influenced by others in formulating your concept of nursing?
   b. How did patients and your friends influence your concept of nursing?
2. Compare the different methods of organizing the staff for giving patient care, drawing on your own experiences.
   a. Have you observed one particular method that seemed to work better than others?
   b. Compare this method to the pure methods of case, functional, team, or primary nursing. How is it the same? How does it differ? What factors in the hospital setting and what factors from the staff have contributed to the success of the method?
3. Interview four nurses from one patient-care unit about their philosophy of nursing practice. How does this philosophy affect patient care?
4. Describe changes in nursing practice that have occurred during the past five years.
   a. What forces created the need for change?
   b. How do you think individual practicing nurses respond to the changes?

5. Abstract three research studies that have been conducted about some phase of nursing practice.
   a. Do you think that practicing nurses have been influenced by these studies?
   b. Do you believe that these studies could be replicated in any nursing setting in a similar way to obtain the same results?
6. Describe four ways that you as a nurse-practitioner influence the organization of nursing service and the improvement of patient care.
7. Evaluate the following objectives:

Patients on bed rest will be provided with a clean, secure environment which protects the patient's safety and meets the patient's needs for comfort. This is accomplished by the following procedures:

(a) Use side rails or restraints (or both) for patients who are confused, comatose, or who have interferences with mobility.
(b) Place beds in low positions to reduce the danger of falling.
(c) Place clean towels, washcloths, soap, and powder in patients' bedside stands, and check the supply daily to ensure that supplies are readily available when needed.
(d) Give patients morning care, which includes elimination, washing hands and face, brushing teeth, combing hair, and other preparation the patient desires for comfort.
(e) Give baths when necessary.
(f) Give passive exercises to patients twice a day for complete range of motion unless contraindicated.
(g) Change patients' positions every two hours.
(h) Place a patient's belongings within reach and remove unnecessary articles from the bedside stands.

   a. Are these objectives clearly stated?
   b. Do these objectives specify a standard of nursing care?
   c. What level of nursing staff (RN, LPN, NA) will find these objectives most useful?

References

1. Corpuz, T. Primary nursing meets needs, expectations of patients and staff. *Hospitals* 51:95, June 1, 1977.
2. Corwin, R. G. Patterns of organizational conflict. *Adm. Sci. Q.* 14:507–520, Dec. 1969.
3. Daeffler, R. J. Patients' perception of care under team and primary nursing. *J. Nurs. Adm.* 5:20–26, 1975.
4. Hackman, J. R. The Designing Work for Individuals and Groups. In J. R. Hackman, E. E. Lawler, and L. W. Porter, *Perspectives on Behavior in Organizations.* New York: McGraw-Hill, 1977. Pp. 242–256.

5. Hall, D. T., and Lawler, E. E.   Job characteristics and pressures and the organizational integration of professionals. *Adm. Sci. Q.* 15:271–281, Sept. 1970.
6. Hall, R. H.   Professionalization and bureaucratization. *Am. Sociol. Rev.* 33:92–103, Feb. 1968.
7. Hall, V. C. *Statutory Regulation of the Scope of Nursing Practice.* Chicago: The Joint Practice Commission, 1975. Pp. 11–35.
8. Hegyvary, S. T. (Ed.)   Symposium on primary nursing. *Nurs. Clin. North Am.* 12:185–186, June 1977.
9. Kase, S., and Swenson, B. *Costs of Hospital-Sponsored Orientation and Inservice Education for Registered Nurses.* USPHS DHEW HRA (77-25) BHM, Division of Nursing, Nov. 1976.
10. Levine, H. D., and Phillip, P. J. *Factors Affecting Staffing Levels and Patterns of Nursing Personnel.* USPHS DHEW HRA (75-6) BHRD, Division of Nursing, Feb. 1975.
11. Marram, G. D., Flynn, K., Abaravich, W., and Carey, S. *Cost-Effectiveness of Primary and Team Nursing.* Wakefield, Mass.: Contemporary Publishing, 1976.
12. Marram, G. D., Schlegel, M. W., and Bevis, O. *Primary Nursing: A Model for Individualized Care.* St. Louis: Mosby, 1974.
13. Nenner, V. C., Curtis, E. M., and Eckoff, C. M.   Primary nursing. *Superv. Nurse,* 8:14–16, May 1977.
14. Werner, J.   The Evanston story: The primary nursing story comes alive. *Nurs. Adm. Q.* 1:9–50, Spring 1977.

Suggested Reading

Abel-Smith, B. *A History of the Nursing Profession.* Atlantic Highlands, N.J.: Humanities Press, 1975.
Anderson, B. E. *Nursing Education in Community Junior Colleges.* Philadelphia: Lippincott, 1966.
Bartels, D., Good, V., and Lampe, S.   The role of the head nurse in primary nursing. *Can. Nurse* 74:26–30, March 1977.
Bliss, A. A., and Cohen, E. D. (Eds.) *The New Health Professionals.* Germantown, Md.: Aspen, 1977.
Brown, B.   The autonomous nurse and primary nursing. *Nurs. Adm. Q.* 1:31–36, Fall 1976.
Brown, E. L. *Nursing Reconsidered: A Study of Change.* Parts 1 and 2. Philadelphia: Lippincott, 1971.
Bullough, B., and Bullough, V. *Expanding Horizons for Nurses.* New York: Springer, 1977.
Campbell, E. B.   The clinical nurse specialist: Joint appointee. *Am. J. Nurs.* 3:543–546, 1970.
Davis, F. *The Nursing Profession: Five Sociological Essays.* New York: Wiley, 1966.
Deloughery, G. L. *History and Trends in Professional Nursing* (8th ed.). St. Louis: Mosby, 1977.

Drexler, A., Yenney, S. L., and Hohman, J. OD: Coping with change. *Hospitals* 51:58–60, Jan. 1, 1977.

Drexler, A., Yenney, S. L., and Hohman, J. OD: An ongoing program. *Hospitals* 51:89–92, Feb. 16, 1977.

Dubos, R. *Man, Medicine and Environment.* New York: Praeger, 1968.

Ellis, B. Nursing profession undergoes intensive scrutiny and adjustment. *Hospitals* 51:139–144, April 1, 1977.

Farrell, N. L., and LaCosta, C. J. Unit administration updated. *Hospitals* 51:75–77, Feb. 16, 1977.

Felton, G. Increasing the quality of nursing care by introducing the concept of primary nursing: A model project. *Nurs. Res.* 24:27–32, Jan./Feb. 1975.

Finer, H. *Administration and the Nursing Services.* New York: Macmillan, 1952.

Georgopoulos, B. S., and Christman, L. The clinical nurse specialist: A role model. *Am. J. Nurs.* 5:1030, 1970.

Goostray, S. *Memoirs: Half a Century in Nursing.* Boston: Nursing Archive, Boston University Mugar Memorial Library, 1969.

Hall, M. B. How do students learn on a primary nursing care unit. *Nurs. Outlook* 25:370–373, June 1977.

Hunnings, V. If you've ever thought about being a nurse-practitioner. *R.N.* 40:35–38, May 1977.

Jennings, C. P. Primary care and the question of obsolescence. *JPN and Mental Health Services* 15:9–17, Jan. 1977.

Jones, D. C., Cooley, P. C., Miedema, A., and Hartwell, T. D. *Trends in RN Supply.* DHEW Publication No. HRA 76-15, Bethesda, Md., March 1976.

Lawrence, R. R. How to deal with resistance to change. *Harvard Bus. Rev.* 1:4, 1969.

Levine, E. What do we know about nurse practitioners? *Am. J. Nurs.* 77:1799–1803, Nov. 1977.

Littlejohn, C. E. From staff nurse to supervisor: A plan of development. *Nurs. Outlook* 24:618–621, Oct. 1976.

Mackay, C., and Ault, L. D. A systematic approach to individualizing nursing care. *J. of Nurs. Adm.* 7:39–48, Jan. 1977.

Mackenzie, R. A. The management process in 3-D. *Harvard Bus. Rev.* 6:67, 1969.

Mager, R. *Preparing Instructional Objectives* (2nd ed.). Palo Alto: Fearon Publishers, 1975.

Miller, M. H., and Flynn, B. C. *Current Perspectives in Nursing Social Issues and Trends.* St. Louis: Mosby, 1977.

Notter, L. E., and Spaulding, E. K. *Professional Nursing Foundations, Perspectives, and Relationships.* (9th ed.) Philadelphia: Lippincott, 1976.

Oda, D. S. Specialized role development: A three-phase process. *Nurs. Outlook* 25:374–377, June 1977.

Ojeda, M. Primary nursing for shortened stay surgical patients. *Superv. Nurse* 7:42, Sept. 1976.

Olesen, V. L., and Whittaker, E. W. *The Silent Dialogue.* San Francisco: Jossey-Bass, 1968.

Redman, B. K. *The Process of Patient Teaching in Nursing* (3rd. ed.). St. Louis: Mosby, 1976.

Rosen, G. *A History of Public Health.* New York: M.D. Publications, 1958.

Schweer, J. E. *Creative Teaching in Clinical Nursing* (2nd ed.). St. Louis: Mosby, 1972.

Simon, H. A. *Administrative Behavior.* New York: Macmillan, 1957.

Sulz, H. A., Zielezny, M., and Kinyon, L. *Longitudinal Study of Nurse Practitioners, Phase I.* USDHEW PHS HRA (76-43), March 1976.

Survey of perceived relationships between chief operating officers and directors of nurses. *Hosp. Top.* 55:38–40, March/April 1977.

The status of continuing education—voluntary and mandatory. *Am. J. Nurs.* 77:410–416, March 1977.

Vollmer, H. M., and Mills, D. L. *Professionalization.* Englewood Cliffs, N.J.: Prentice-Hall, 1966.

Walker, V. H. *Nursing and Ritualistic Practice.* New York: Macmillan, 1967.

Winstead-Fry, P. The need to differentiate a nursing self. *Am. J. Nurs.* 77:1452–1454, Sept. 1977.

4. Group Leadership in Nursing Management

All nurses are managers by virtue of their professional status. They manage patient care wherever they work—as school nurses, as industrial nurses, or as hospital staff nurses. Whether the nurse works alone or with others, the dimension of management is present in the work situation. The nurse works in a social climate in which both the care process and the management process require leadership and working with groups. Both of these topics, leadership and working with groups, will be explored in this chapter.

Leadership in the Organizational Structure

Health-care agencies vary considerably in the way nursing staffs are organized. Nurses are often given management responsibilities that include management both of patient care and of personnel with less educational preparation, such as licensed practical or vocational nurses and nurse's aides. In some agencies this dual role is well defined for the nursing staff. In others there may be no definite structure that delineates the scope of managerial responsibility.

Consider the patient-care units in hospitals you are familiar with. Do these units have appointed team leaders or their equivalents? Or do the units have rotating team leaders so that the responsibilities of managing are given to different persons on different days? Are management functions the sole responsibility of the head nurse? Or are clinical specialists given responsibility for managing patient care? You may be able to cite different organizational structures among different hospitals and in the same hospital.

Functions required of nurses for managing people are determined to some extent by organizational structures, the number of nurses employed to care for a given number of patients, by the qualifications (both experience and education) of the staff members, and by the supporting staff employed for a unit, such as ward or unit managers.

True management of patient care by a leader is possible only if he or she fills an appointed position. This management implies working toward long-term goals. In order to achieve the goals of patient care over a period of time, one must work consistently with people and the resources through a process of growth and expansion toward achieving. Demands for creative and innovative nursing can be met only by continual application of the management process.

What happens if there is no designated manager in the organizational structure? When nurses rotate in management positions, the staff expends energy adapting to the style of management employed by each different person. Managers tend to focus on events that occur during their time as managers. When this period is just one or two days, it is difficult not only to determine long-range goals but also to concentrate on achieving such goals. The short-term manager places emphasis on daily events rather than on the growth of staff members over time. The manager by the day is actually a troubleshooter rather than a progressive planner.

DEVELOPMENT OF THE STUDENT NURSE AS A MANAGER

The variability among health-care agencies and their expectations of nurses makes it confusing for a beginning nurse to define clearly what a nurse-manager's role ought to be. The beginning nurse is also going through one of the most difficult career transitions—that of becoming a manager. Although student nurses gradually assume the stature required of nurses for managing patient care in their educational programs, they often find that functioning as an employee in the work situation is quite different from being a student in a guided learning experience.

Students first learn management through learning how to organize the very basic aspects of patient care, such as giving baths, ambulating patients, providing for proper diet, and giving medications. As the student progresses through the educational program, more complex functions are mastered so that eventually the student can successfully care for a critically or chronically ill patient, managing many different but related events which affect the patient. Educational programs are developed sequentially to broaden the nurse's scope of knowledge about patient care. During the educational process the student becomes increasingly confident of his or her ability to handle difficult situations. And yet, it is normal for a student to feel confident about student experiences but insecure about the expectations of employment as a registered nurse. Despite the fact that the basic expectations of patients for nursing care are no different for the student than for the graduate, the student often perceives that this scope of functions has changed overnight following graduation.

A "first job" as a registered nurse is a new and different experience. A beginning nurse perceives employment as a challenge or test of competency. The challenge can be met with either anticipation, apprehension, or both, depending on one's degree of self-confidence.

One major difference between being a student and being employed is that the beginning nurse is expected to assume a leadership position in the work situation and to interact with all personnel as a professional nurse who influences the behavior of others. Responsibilities in this interaction are inherently different from those required of a student. The student usually focuses on the health care of a particular patient or a small group of patients; as an employee, the graduate nurse is part of an organization and must focus on both patient care and working with the staff.

LEADERSHIP ABILITIES

What is the difference between being a leader and being a manager? Leadership is closely associated with management. Every manager does not necessarily have to be a leader. In nursing, however, where the work is accomplished by working with people, leadership is emphasized as a necessary qualification of nurse-managers. Defining leadership as the ability to influence the behavior of others is an oversimplification because leadership depends on the leader, the group being led, and the situation in which leadership takes place.

Compare two leaders: Mary is a good nurse who can be described as essentially task-oriented—that is, she pays attention to detail and is precise in carrying out the tasks of nursing; she likes structure and functions best in a well-defined situation with definite tasks to perform. Jane, on the other hand, is restless and thrives on change; she also is a good nurse and prefers situations which are unstructured so that she can make decisions that are flexible. Each of these leaders presents a different personality. Mary will be a successful leader in a structured situation that defines her role, whereas Jane would not be a successful leader in a structured situation—she would probably try to change the structure to meet her need for variety and change. Similarly, Mary would not be considered a good leader in an unstructured situation.

FACTORS AFFECTING SELECTION OF A LEADER

As you can see, leadership is effective if the leader's personality and abilities are matched to the requirements of a given situation. Because health-care agencies are variable in their philosophies, structures, and concomitant expectations for nurses, what constitutes a good leader for one might not for another. For this reason, the leadership abilities of a given nurse must be considered in relation to the needs of the situation.

Because leadership is so important to management in nursing, the choice of an appointed manager often depends on an individual's leadership abilities. These abilities can include the nurse's knowledge of patient care, natural or acquired leadership abilities, and familiarity with the organization. The importance of each of these factors in choosing a manager depends on the particular situation. Let us explore each separately.

Knowledge is often called a corollary of power. In nursing, knowledge enables the nurse to make decisions that other staff members may not be qualified to make or may be hesitant to make for themselves. The nurse with the most nursing expertise tends to be recognized by the group as a natural leader in matters related to making decisions about patient care. This is evidenced when staff members who need support or assistance in giving such care seek help from the nurse with the most knowledge. This nurse is often appointed to a formal leadership position when expertise is the most important criterion.

Natural or acquired leadership abilities are usually evidenced by the nurse's ability to work cooperatively with other staff members. This person tends to emerge as a natural leader because he or she can influence the behavior of others through personality. This type of leader can make others feel understood and important, usually has a good sense of humor, and can make other people feel satisfied with themselves and accepted by the group. The ability to work well with others is an important criterion for selection of a leader when group cohesiveness is a primary factor in the choice.

Familiarity with the organization is important for a leader in situations that require knowledge of the organization's policies and procedures. Although nurses adjust to the expectations of an organization at different rates, they are usually not secure in their understanding of the working relationships in an organization until they have worked there for some time. In situations in which the leader must be familiar with the operating policies of the organization, the nurse with tenure is usually appointed to the leadership position. Some organizations traditionally promote from "within the ranks" rather than selecting people from the "outside" for leadership positions.

INTERACTION WITH GROUP MEMBERS

Another, perhaps more complicated way of exploring leadership of nurses centers on the role of the nurse in interaction with all persons involved in giving patient care. These people include the patient, family or friends, the nursing staff, and other medical personnel, who contribute to patient care. The nurse-manager's interaction influences the effectiveness of patient care, which depends on coordination of the efforts of many persons. Being able to influence a group is a function of leadership.

CLASSIFICATION OF INTERACTING GROUPS

Fiedler [1] has classified the leader's interaction with group members according to the amount of power and influence a leader exerts in an organization. His classification of interacting groups includes three factors: (1) position power, (2) the structure of the task, and (3) the interpersonal relationship between the leader and group members. His theory can be adapted to nursing leadership.

Position Power. The first factor cited, position power, can be related to the nurse's sanctioned role for giving patient care. The knowledge which qualifies the nurse to become a professional gives the nurse the authority to be a leader in the nurse-patient relationship. If the patient accepts the position power of the nurse, it can be said that the nurse has high position power. However, if the patient's perception of the status and role expectations of the nurse negates the nurse's authority, the nurse has low position power in the nurse-patient relationship.

An appointed manager is given a legitimate position in an organizational structure. When a nurse is appointed to the position of team or modular leader, for example, that nurse is given authority for leading a group of staff members by the organization. This appointed position gives the nurse power to guide, direct, and control the activities of staff members. The amount of power given the leader to control staff activities affects the interaction between the staff and the leader. The group tends to comply with the leader's direction when the position is supported by organizational authority. For example, if the staff knows that the leader's evaluation of a staff member's performance is important when salary increases are considered, that leader will probably have high position power.

Position power in an organization must also be associated with the leader's ability to gain the group's cooperation. A leader's position power is visibly lower when staff members do not accept the leader.

Position power can give only formal authority. In an organization this formal authority can be negated if informal leaders exert more influence on the group than does the appointed leader.

Structure of the Task. When a group of people are involved in performance of work, the second factor in the classification system, the structure of the task, is important. The total task of administering patient care can be viewed as all of the work that must be accomplished to achieve the purpose of health care. The work of giving patient care is often divided among the many leaders. Tasks assigned to leaders encompass defining goals, organizing care, activating the care plans, controlling care given, and evaluating the work. Because these tasks are broad and general, they are complex and unstructured.

In comparison, nurse's aides are assigned the technical aspects of patient care that are well defined and can be structured. The need for task structure decreases as the staff member's knowledge, experience, and sanctioned authority increase. Tasks for a licensed practical nurse require less structure than those for a nurse's aide. A registered nurse requires less task structure than the licensed practical nurse. The ability to understand concepts and to make decisions are important criteria in determining the structure required for group members.

In nursing, the leader's tasks vary according to the capabilities of staff members. If the staff includes nurse's aides, licensed practical or vocational nurses, and a few professional nurses, the leader's tasks will include making detailed, clearly stated, and well-structured assignments. These assignments must be more definitive and must be accompanied by support and guidance because the needs of the staff members are more specific. The leader in this instance assumes the major responsibility for defining and helping others work toward achieving long-term goals.

When the nursing staff comprises more professional nurses than subprofessionals, the tasks must be assigned so that the professional nurses have an opportunity to use their conceptual abilities for defining and directing patient care. Tasks for professional staff members are broader, more general, more flexible, and unstructured. In this instance, the leader's tasks also are unstructured and complex, and would probably revolve around provision for continuing growth for staff members, development of methods for group decision-making, and participation in defining and achieving long-term goals for improvement of patient care.

Interaction of the Leader with Staff Members. In both situations just described, interaction is important. When working with nonprofessionals, the interaction depends on the leader's ability to define expectations in specific terms, to give specific directions, and to provide support, encouragement, and assistance in giving patient care. In comparison, the leader's interaction with a professional staff is based on the leader's ability to allow each person freedom to practice nursing autonomously according to his or her prerogative for giving care while coordinating the efforts of all staff members for achieving goals of patient care.

These differences in interaction stem from the fact that professionals share a common knowledge of patient care and have the same social sanction and legal authority for giving care. The major difference between professional nurse staff members and the professional nurse-leader is the leader's organizational authority. Professionals do not depend on the leader to direct the giving of patient care. When working with professionals, therefore, the leader must exert a positive influence toward their work satisfaction and development as practitioners. The leader of a group of subprofessional staff members must exert positive influence toward their growth and satisfaction but also exerts more control over the activities of the group in the performance of the work. Certain aspects of nursing care can be broken down into procedures and routines that can be assigned with specificity and that can be performed effectively by persons who do not fully understand the implications of their work. However, this can be accomplished only if the leader provides professional direction and makes decisions about care.

Acceptance of the leader by the group is paramount. The leader who is appointed to a position and who is capable of handling the complex tasks required of a leader must also be accepted by group members to be effective. Acceptance by group members is augmented by the formal appointment of the leader by the organization, because it implies that the organization will support the leader's authority by defining the role expectations of the leader and by supporting the leader's decisions as he or she functions in the designated role.

Recognition of this authority is sometimes demonstrated by patients who ask for the head nurse or supervisor when they have questions because they know that these persons have more authority than other staff members. These patients believe that the head nurse or supervisor has more knowledge and more power to "get things done." In a similar manner the physician might tell a modular leader about a specific patient's care because the leader has the responsibility and authority to direct other staff members in the patient's care. The physician believes that the leader will make sure that the staff understands the communication. Communications directed to the leader from all sources in the work situation increase the leader's information and understanding of events related to patient care so that decisions will be more effective. This information is necessary for coordination of staff members' work.

Can you remember the first time you were a team or modular leader? Did staff members tell you about the progress of their patients' care and about the problems they were having? Did you find that as an appointed leader you were the recipient of much information you might not have received otherwise? Because of this flow of information to the appointed leader, one often hears the comment "I really like to be leader because I get to know what is going on," or "I did not realize that being a leader was so involved." These comments demonstrate the fact that people in an organization tend to follow patterns of behavior and prescribed pathways for communication. They accept appointed leaders because they have definite role expectations of appointed leaders.

LEADERSHIP STUDIES
The fact still remains that some leaders are more effective than others. What are the attributes of successful leaders? Over the years, many people have attempted to define leadership, but a clear definition of leadership remains elusive. Early leadership studies were concerned with attempts to isolate characteristics or traits that leaders have in common. One of the problems of using this approach is that the findings of one study often cannot be replicated in others. Leaders who have been studied do not demonstrate common or consistent traits or characteristics. However, a few characteristics do seem to be applicable to most leaders. For example, studies conducted by the University of Minnesota indicate that leaders are highly motivated, tend to be more educated than others, and are more intelligent [8]. Ghiselli [2] has recently found that leaders tend to be independent, be involved in activities, like intensive thinking, enjoy working with others as leader, and take some risks. It is interesting to note that people can have many different types of personalities and yet still have these characteristics.

Studies that approached leadership from the aspect of leader behaviors followed early research concerned with leadership traits. The classic Ohio State University studies [7, 9] were concerned with defining the types of leadership behaviors and their effects on workers' performance and level of satisfaction. Two independent factors of leader behavior that were found to increase both performance and satisfaction are consideration and initiating structure. Consideration behaviors include trust, respect, friendship, and warmth. Initiating structure behaviors refer to the leader's ability to define and to accomplish the work through others.

Another classic set of studies was conducted by theorists at the University of Michigan [6]. Results of these studies indicate that the higher producing leaders spend more time planning and less time conducting task operations and that they give workers more latitude. Two of these theorists, Katz and Kahn [6], also demonstrated that supervisors used different styles, close supervision and general supervision. General supervision, in which workers are allowed more latitude, was thought to be more effective. Other research studies have indicated, however, that close supervision can also result in increased productivity in certain situations.

A number of studies have been conducted to investigate the influence of the situation on leadership. These studies include Fiedler's contingency theory [1]. This theory was developed retrospectively from accumulated data, and some experts feel that this method is not highly credible. The contingency theory developed by Fiedler is useful, however, in describing leadership. The contingency theory indicates that the effects of leadership are contingent on group outcomes. The leader behaviors are effective if the worker's performance achieves the desired outcomes. In this theory, the leader's needs, the nature of the work group, and the situation are considered to be interrelated in determining the effectiveness of the leader in achieving performance outcomes.

The path-goal theory of leadership initially authored by House [4] is somewhat similar to Fiedler's theories. This theory was also developed from retrospective evaluation of data. The path-goal theory includes four major styles of leadership: directive, supportive, participative, and achievement-oriented. The leader is viewed as one who supplements the work environment by providing aspects such as guidance, support, and rewards that are not otherwise present in the environment. This theory takes into account the nature of the situation, the worker's needs and goals, and the leader's ability to use power and to stimulate motivation.

The path-goal theory of leadership is based on the concept that workers will be motivated to accomplish the work if they believe that their efforts will lead to rewards and that rewards will be given for effort. The basis for the worker's motivation includes a number of factors: the worker's internal satisfactions, which are related to self-actualization; the external satisfactions provided by the organization, such as status and pay; the clarity of goals that indicate what is expected; and clear statements of the rewards that will be achieved. An effective leader "clears the path" to goal achievement by removing impediments in the worker's path, by clearly defining the path, by providing rewards throughout the work cycle to foster continued worker motivation, and by ensuring that effort is rewarded as the worker expected by giving rewards for achievement.

Another approach to the study of leadership is to define the functions of leadership that are required to maintain the workers and to promote productivity. Two types of functions, expressive and instrumental, have been defined. Expressive functions are geared to the social and emotional aspects of the workers' interaction and are geared toward "maintaining" the workers. Instrumental functions are task-oriented, such as providing resources and defining tasks that are necessary for production of work. It has been postulated that one person cannot always perform both instrumental and expressive functions effectively since the focus of these two functions is quite different. It could be that one person is required to maintain the work group and another to ensure performance.

As studies of leadership have evolved, there is increasing evidence that organizational behavior is complex and that different types of leaders can be equally effective. Since there is no clear definition of leadership, the beginning leader often develops a leadership style through trial and error, learning through experiences. The beginning leader will probably be most effective if he or she accepts the role of "leader" and then develops a style of leadership that is an expression of his or her personality.

Working with Groups
There are many instances in which certain types of work in nursing are accomplished in groups. Participation in groups enables people to use their leadership talents through interaction with other group members. The leader who works with groups can use this interaction to develop competency of group members and to stimulate their motivation to produce. Gibb [3] has written that ". . . viewed in

relation to the individual, leadership is not an attribute of the personality but a quality of his role within a particular and specified social system." When people become involved in groups they take on roles within the group. These roles are factors in the effectiveness of the group interaction and personalities of members are subsumed to these roles. In the following section we will explore some characteristics of groups in the work situation.

PURPOSE AND PROCESS OF GROUP INTERACTION

Groups of people work together in organizations to accomplish work. In nursing, certain patterns of care delivery, such as team nursing or modular nursing, use job designs in which groups are an integral part of the design. Groups are also used in management for a number of different purposes. Task forces and project groups are examples of specially assigned groups that serve a particular purpose. Committees are another example of how groups are used in organizations to coordinate effort and to promote communication. These committees can be standing committees or ad hoc committees that deal with matters important to the organization.

Nurses also work in groups to give patient care. These groups may include other nurses, medically related personnel such as doctors and therapists, and the patient, family, or friends who participate in the care-giving process. These people may meet in conferences to plan care, evaluate care, solve operational problems, coordinate functions of a number of different people, and develop new ideas about care delivery. Groups may be used for providing instruction for staff or for patients. Interaction of people in groups is an aspect of working with others in an organization. Groups provide a medium through which some of the work of an organization is accomplished.

Groups can have many different purposes, but the processes of group interaction follow a sequence: developing strategy, setting goals, working out problems, defining methods for achieving goals, implementing the group decisions, and terminating the activity. Every group is different not only because purposes are different, but also because the group membership is different. To be effective in leading a group, the leader clearly defines the purpose of the group, determines the qualifications and concomitant contributions of the members, and applies concepts of group process to developing effective interaction among members.

Let us consider some concepts of group process that can be applied to working with a group of staff nurses. If the group works together continuously, group process can be used to promote learning so that staff members increase knowledge and competency in giving patient care through group interaction. A stable and cohesive group of staff members can promote growth through continuous participation in progressively more complex group activities. This growth is enhanced by stability of group membership. When staff members shift from group to group, long-term group activities are thwarted. Have you experienced attending a group meeting one week in which the members organized, defined purposes and goals, and approved group decisions, returning the following week to find new members whose ideas completely changed decisions made at the first meeting? This experience illustrates how shifting group membership thwarts progress toward goal achievement by group members.

Groups deal with both content and process. The content is the purpose of the group or the group's task structure. The process is the way that the group members interact with each other in dealing with the content. Staff members often use the group process to meet individual needs, and the leader who recognizes these individual needs can foster group interaction that enables members to meet their own needs while also accomplishing the group tasks. The leader's task is to prevent loss of effort expended in process so that the group will be productive in accomplishing its tasks.

MOTIVATION TO JOIN A GROUP

An initial activity that helps the group leader recognize individual needs of members is to find out why each member has become part of the group. Answers to questions such as Why is Betty working as a nurse's aide? or Why does Bonnie travel an hour each day to work when she could be employed as a licensed practical nurse in a hospital much closer to her home? or Why has Rita elected to work in this particular unit? often give the leader clues to the staff member's basic motivation to working in the organization. This motivation influences the level of the worker's involvment in the staff's group activities for improving patient care.

The leader uses this information about the staff member's motivation to structure group tasks. If the staff is highly motivated to achieve the group purposes, the leader can immediately structure the tasks to achieve these purposes. If the members are not highly motivated to achieve group tasks, however, the leader structures the group tasks in such a way that the members' personal interests are challenged. Initial tasks for this group can be centered on improving some aspect of the work situation that involves all of the members. Successful completion of a task such as arranging coffee-break times helps the group members to develop a sense of "ownership" for group membership that will help the leader introduce tasks geared to improving patient care.

Forming a cohesive group contributes to the productivity of a group. Ivancevich, Szilagyi, and Wallace [5] cite factors that increase group cohesiveness as "(1) agreement on group goals, (2) frequency of interaction, (3) personal attractiveness, (4) intergroup competition, and (5) favorable evaluation." Common goals serve to bind the group members together and frequency of interaction also promotes a feeling of closeness. When group members enjoy working with one another, are in competition with other groups, and when they perceive that their performance as a member of a group is rewarded, cohesiveness is increased. On the other hand these authors cite "disagreement on goals, large groups, unpleasant group experiences, competition within the group, and domination of one or more group members" as factors that decrease cohesiveness. The group leader can also develop a sense of trust among group members by clearly defining their roles. The leader outlines the boundaries of group decision-making and informs the members of the degree of authority and freedom they have in developing group activities. This authority and freedom stem from the organizational policies and structure, as well as from the capabilities of the group members. In defining the latitude for decision-making, the group leader must discern the level of task that the group members can realistically handle. Definition of roles and of the latitude the group has for decision-making reduces confusion and helps the group focus on the group tasks.

Acceptance of Group Members. Another way the leader contributes to group members' security is through acceptance of each person in the group. Acceptance can be demonstrated when the leader seeks information and opinions from group members and then visibly uses the information. Courtesy and respect for others can be sensed by group members, and this influences their response to the leader. Thus, the leader sets the tone for group interaction. Members usually want to be accepted not only by the leader but also by others in the group. Positive relationships among group members contribute to the effectiveness of the group. Knowledge that members accept an individual, even though that person's ideas are not always accepted, enhances the member's security in the group.

Group members' needs to achieve vary, and their requirements for help from one another when giving patient care also vary. Staff members can attain need satisfaction by participating in group activities and can share expertise and assistance in giving care with other group members.

EFFECTIVE GROUP INTERACTION

The need for acceptance by others may have to be dealt with before an individual can participate in a group. The leader's recognition of individual differences, encouragement of freedom of expression, and support for all staff members set the tone for interaction. How does the leader accomplish all of this? How do group members contribute to this? Let us consider a group:

Mary, Ruby, Bonnie, and Sam are meeting to discuss a particular patient's care. Mary cannot concentrate because she is bothered by the way Bonnie slumps in her chair. Mary finally tells Bonnie that her "slumping posture" bothers her. Mary then feels better, even though Bonnie may not change her position. Bonnie can react to Mary's comment in a number of ways. If she is secure in the group, she may respond with a laughing comment. She may even attempt to sit up. If she is not secure, she will probably react with a defensive comment, or she might withdraw from participation in the group.

In the situation just described, the leader may intervene by commenting that Bonnie may slump, but she really knows a lot about the particular patient's medications. More secure members of the group may also intervene. They may in a future meeting make a point of talking openly about individual differences in an effort to demonstrate to Mary that other members are accepted despite their personal idiosyncrasies. Openness about individual differences can be an adjunct to group participation. Familiarity with an object or a person, unless that object or person is continually fear-provoking, usually increases one's security.

Encouragement of Free Expression. Understanding of one another also fosters free expression for group members. The leader who allows free expression can determine how staff members perceive nursing and how they view their roles in giving patient care by interpreting what they say. Expressing ideas gives group members an opportunity to get acquainted with one another and with the leader. How does the leader allow free expression?

First of all, the leader must be both a good listener and patient. Let us say that in a group meeting Ruby makes a statement that the leader knows is incorrect. Instead of saying, "No, Ruby, you are wrong," the leader should wait to hear what other members of the group say. Mary, for example, may agree with Ruby, but Sam and Bonnie may explain why the statement is incorrect. When the correct definition emerges from group discussion, this definition is accepted more readily by all group members. Usually, if given freedom, the group will arrive at the right definition, because people can change their opinions and ideas through discussion. The leader should intervene only if the group does not correct Ruby's statement, or if asked by the group to intervene.

If the leader responds by saying, "No, Ruby, you are wrong," the group will probably be affected in a negative way. Ruby may be very hesitant to speak again. When others see what has happened to Ruby, they also may guard their comments so that they say what the leader will accept. The group members assume important roles in helping the group achieve through their interaction.

Individual Roles in the Group. Roles of group members are usually naturally assumed. Mary, for example, may have a natural facility for expanding ideas. Sam may excel in clarifying what the group is saying. Bonnie may be the accepted information giver, and Ruby may stimulate the group to stay on the topic. The members' responsibility for the group then fits with the personality and abilities of each. Through group interaction these roles are accepted so that the group is really controlled by its members.

Some of the roles that group members assume include initiating, information seeking, information giving, clarifying, summarizing, gate-keeping, standard setting, and mediating. The initiator is one who introduces new concepts or ideas. The information seeker questions group members about facts or data that relate to the group's task. The information giver presents these facts or data. Clarification is the role of the person who interprets the ideas of group members and who tends to intervene when there is confusion. The person who summarizes synthesizes ideas presented to lead to a conclusion. The gatekeeper is one who encourages free participation of group members, and the standard setter focuses the group members' attention on the goals or standards to be achieved. The mediator attempts to resolve conflict or disagreement and intervenes when tension among group members develops. These roles are aspects of group behavior that allow the group members to deal productively with both the processes of their interaction and the task to be accomplished.

Peer Group Pressure. When belonging to a group becomes important for staff members, the norms of the group help to control behavior of those who tend to impede group process. This is called peer group pressure. A person who finds that deflating another's ego is met with group rejection will usually cease such action. A person who might ordinarily try to block the group discussion will try to cooperate if belonging to the group is more important than the personal need to be an obstructionist.

Peer pressure can be facilitating or detrimental to a group. The established behavioral norms of group members affect not only the members' interaction but also the types of choices that the group makes. When dealing with tasks, the group determines strategies that represent the choices of the group members. When the function of the group is to develop innovative approaches to patient care, the behavioral norms of the members may hinder consideration of new or different ideas. This is particularly true when group members have fixed ideas about patient care that have not changed over time. These members may be unable to choose strategies for the group task that are representative of current or changing nursing practice. The group leader must make an effort to help the group members develop new behavioral norms and endeavors to guide the group to the level of the most competent member. When the group leader is working to change behavioral norms, group effort is used in process activities that lead to development of new concepts and ideas. This process may necessarily precede actively working on the task, thereby lengthening the time required to accomplish goals.

COMMON UNDERSTANDING OF GOALS

As stated earlier, the group interaction is the vehicle for achieving group purposes. Once the group determines its working relationships, it can define and accept the purpose of work to be accomplished. A group of nursing staff members is a continuous group because its purposes are never terminated. Therefore, it is important that the leader organize group tasks so that segments of each task can be completed while also ensuring that there is always something new to work toward. Why? Because completing something gives satisfaction, but having no purpose leads to disinterest. Without a purpose the group may consider staff meetings a waste of time. The leader must stimulate interest by continually stretching the group to new challenges.

How does the leader determine where to begin in defining a group purpose in the maze of problems that can be recognized in almost every nursing situation? Members will become involved more readily in a group if its activities are relevant to their personal concerns. If group members are given the opportunity to discuss problems they consider important, the leader can focus their attention on the most prominent problem. Group activity can then center on working for something definite that is pertinent to group members.

When discussing pertinent concerns of group members, the leader should understand that a common understanding of goals depends on a common definition of words used to express these goals. The processes of clarifying, interpreting, and expanding ideas are continuous as the group works together. Most words can be interpreted in numerous ways. For this reason, definition of terms should emerge from interaction among members so that everyone in the group has a common understanding.

DETERMINING REALISTIC GOALS
Knowledge about the staff members' abilities and capabilities and about the goals for patient care helps the leader determine realistic goals for the group activities. The leader with a predetermined plan for the group's function will be more likely to achieve desired results, even if the predetermined plan is changed by the group. This predetermined plan helps the leader maintain direction and provides task structure for the group's interaction. Considerations for developing this plan include the knowledge and experience of group members and their capability for organizing their thoughts for planning. New, inexperienced nurse's aides need to be given well-defined problems for solution if they are to participate effectively in the group, whereas experienced aides who are familiar with nursing terminology and care probably need less structure. Defining problems for group interaction that the members can solve prevents frustration for both the members and the leader.

For example, a group may be totally overwhelmed if the leader presents an activity such as writing objectives for patient care. The leader must present the activity to the staff members in terms that are understood and in a form that the staff members can handle. Instead of asking the staff to write objectives, the leader might ask them to consider what they would list as important for patient care if they were the patients. The leader can then translate the ideas expressed by the staff into statements of objectives. The leader actually supplements that portion or segment of the activity that the staff is not able to accomplish.

GROUP PROCESS IN MANAGEMENT

In order to determine what segment of an activity the staff is able to accomplish, the leader must have a concept of all components of a given activity. This is comparable to the way a leader assigns care according to the abilities of staff members. When ideas come from the staff members, the leader must determine their feasibility and, if they are relevant, put them to use. Sometimes the leader may incorporate an idea into an already existing plan or into channels that will be acceptable for the organization. A leader sets limits for exploring ideas so that staff members can use their energies to make plans that will be workable and acceptable to eveyone affected by the idea and its implications. If the idea means a change in the way services are coordinated in an existing plan, the leader must "clear the idea" with other personnel involved.

Following clear definition of the work the group is to accomplish, the group must consistently work for results. A guide to activities which lead to results through group action is outlined as follows. Notice how ideas can be translated into group activities.

I-dentification of problems.
D-efinition of goals for patient care.
E-ngrossment in resource information, facts, principles, concepts.
A-nalysis of information.
S-ynthesis of ideas for formulating a plan which can be activated and evaluated.

This demonstrates how the group can become involved in the management process. When staff members participate in formulation of methods for improving patient care, they need support and encouragement from the manager. Throughout the group process of working out problems and reaching a conclusion to activities, the leader helps the group realize that progress must be planned, that it takes effort, and that sometimes results are achieved slowly. When group process is used in management, members of the group need to be continually informed of their progress, and they will be increasingly motivated to participate if results are achieved. The support of the leader must also be continuous. Knowing when to intervene in group interaction by making an authoritative statement, and how to intervene in matters external to the group that affect its progress are management responsibilities.

CONCLUSIONS

If the group works effectively, the leader can expect to find that group members become increasingly sensitive to one another, that they are more accepting of individual differences, that they learn by sharing information and ideas, and that the group is capable of achieving results that each person would find difficult to achieve by working alone. An objective of management is to help workers achieve their potential by growing through performance of work. In nursing, when staff members continually grow, they give better patient care.

Study Questions

1. Susan is a personable, attractive nurse who is sensitive to other people's feelings. She has a good sense of humor which enables her to help other nursing personnel relax. Susan is well liked, and she is always able to get other staff members to help her with her work. Mary is an efficient nurse who has worked in the agency for six years. She always knows answers to questions about policies, where to get equipment and supplies, and whom to call when problems arise. Joseph is often called a "walking encyclopedia" by other nursing personnel. He knows what to do in unusual or emergency nursing situations. His ability for making diagnoses is superior to that of the other nurses, and he is often called on as a consultant by other nurses. Choose one of these nurses and explain why that person would be the best leader.
2. Consider the nurses you know. Choose the one you think is the best leader.
   a. Explain why you think this person is the best leader.
   b. What outstanding qualities does this person have?
   c. Describe the situation in which this person leads.
   d. How does this person influence other people?
3. Describe your own style of leadership.
   a. What types of nursing situations do you prefer?
   b. How do you work with other personnel?
   c. Are you able to influence others?
   d. Is your knowledge of nursing sufficient to allow you to work with other personnel as a leader?
   e. Is your knowledge of nursing good enough to allow you to be creative in planning patient care?

Group Session

1. Meet with your group members and talk about the major problems you recognize in giving patient care. (This should be a brainstorming session which is free and open for all members.)
2. Record the most frequently mentioned problems. Analyze them to determine whether they are related problems and whether the group can realistically become involved in solving them.
3. Identify how these problems are influenced by:
   a. The patients
   b. The staff
   c. The organization of nursing care
   d. The health-care agency organization
4. Check your summary of expressed problems with what actually happens on the unit by recording the major problems which occur each day for four consecutive days. Do the problems expressed by the staff occur consistently? How do the working relationships of staff members contribute to these problems?
5. Choose the problem you feel is outstanding, and work with the group for its solution. Define the limits of the group and of the problem so that group members know what is expected of them.
6. As the group works together consider the following:
   a. Do group members accept one another?
   b. Do group members express their thoughts freely?
   c. Does the group define terms for common understanding?
7. Observe each group member's interaction and describe the roles that each person assumes.
   a. Initiator
   b. Information seeker
   c. Information giver
   d. Clarifier
   e. Summarizer
   f. Gatekeeper
   g. Standard setter
   h. Mediator

References

1. Fiedler, F. E. *A Theory of Leadership Effectiveness.* New York: McGraw-Hill, 1967.
2. Ghiselli, E. E. The validity of management traits related to occupational level. *Pers. Psychol.* 16:109, 1963.
3. Gibb, C. The Principles and Traits of Leadership. In C. G. Browne and T. S. Cohn (Eds.), *The Study of Leadership* (2nd ed.). Danville, Ill.: Interstate Printers and Publishers, 1958.
4. House, R. J. A path-goal theory of leader effectiveness. *Adm. Sci. Q.* 16:321, 1971.
5. Ivancevich, J. M., Szilagyi, A. D., and Wallace, M. J. *Organizational Behavior and Performance.* Santa Monica, Calif.: Goodyear Publishing, 1977.

6. Katz, D., and Kahn, R. L.   Leadership Practices in Relation to Productivity and Morale. In D. Cartwright and A. Zander (Eds.), *Group Dynamics*. Evanston, Ill.: Row, Peterson, 1960.
7. Lowin, A. E., Hrapchak, W. J., and Kavanagh, M. J.   Consideration and initiating structure: An experimental investigation of leadership traits. *Adm. Sci. Q.* 14:239, 1969.
8. Luthans, F.   *Organizational Behavior* (2nd ed.). New York: McGraw-Hill, 1977. Pp. 434–466.
9. Schriesheim, C., and Kerr, S.   Psychometric properties of the Ohio State leadership scales. *Psychol. Bull.* 81:756, 1974.

Suggested Reading

Barrett, J.   *The Head Nurse and Her Changing Role* (3rd ed.). New York: Appleton-Century-Crofts, 1975.

Behling, O., and Schriesheim, C.   *Organizational Behavior Theory and Research Application*. Boston: Allyn & Bacon, 1976.

Bowers, D. G.   *Systems of Organization*. Ann Arbor: University of Michigan Press, 1976.

Browne, C. G., and Cohn, T. S.   *The Study of Leadership* (2nd ed.). Danville, Ill.: Interstate Printers and Publishers, 1958.

Claus, K. E., and Bailey, J. T.   *Power and Influence in Health Care: A New Approach to Leadership*. St. Louis: Mosby, 1977.

Day, R. C., and Hamblin, R. L.   Some effects of close and punitive styles of leadership. *Am. J. Sociol.* 69:499, 1964.

Ginzberg, E.   *The Development of Human Resources*. New York: McGraw-Hill, 1966.

Grissum, M., and Spengler, C.   *Womanpower and Health Care*. Boston: Little, Brown, 1976.

Gruendemann, B. J.   Preoperative group sessions part of nursing process. *AORN* 26:257–262, Aug. 1977.

Hackman, J. R., and Morris, C. G.   Improving Group Performance Effectiveness. In J. R. Hackman, E. E. Lawler, and L. W. Porter (Eds.), *Perspectives on Behavior in Organizations*. New York: McGraw-Hill, 1977.

Herzberg, F.   One more time: How do you motivate employees? *Harvard Bus. Rev.* 1:53, 1968.

Likert, R., and Likert, J. G.   *New Ways of Managing Conflict*. New York: McGraw-Hill, 1976.

Mager, R. F., and Beach, K. M.   *Developing Vocational Instruction*. Palo Alto: Fearon Publishers, 1967.

Maier, N. R. F.   *Problem Solving and Creativity in Individuals and Groups*. Belmont, Cal.: Brooks/Cole, 1970.

Merton, R. K.   The social nature of leadership. *Am. J. Nurs.* 12:2614, 1969.

Nelson, M.   Building a better team. *Nursing '77* 7:65–68, July 1977.

Pollak, G. K.   *Leadership of Discussion Groups*. New York: Spectrum Publications (Wiley), 1975.

Roche, W. J., and MacKinnon, N. L.   Motivating people with meaningful work. *Harvard Bus. Rev.* 3:97, 1970.

Stevens, B. J. (Ed.)   The delicate art of nursing supervision and leadership. *Nurs. Dig.* 5:9–13, Fall 1977.

Szilagyi, A. D., and Sims, H. P.   An exploration of the path-goal theory of leadership in a health-care facility. *Acad. Manage. J.* 17:622, Dec. 1974.

Webber, R. A. *Management: Basic Elements of Managing Organizations.* Homewood, Ill.: Irwin, 1975.

5. Management for Quality Patient Care

Controlling is a management process that incorporates all other processes associated with management. Controlling can be viewed as the essence of management since it is concerned with ensuring that an organization is productive. In this chapter we will explore some basic issues of controlling and will describe two of the mangement processes used to control the productivity in an organization, quality assurance programs and budgeting.

Organizational Control

Current health-care literature contains much information about quality assurance programs. Such programs are evolving as a result of the federal government's involvement in health care. Laws such as Medicare, Medicaid, and the PSRO legislation (PL 92-603) contain provisions for measuring certain aspects of care. The PSRO legislation mandates that there be both certification of need on the patient's admission and continued review of care, evaluation of medical care, and analysis of the patient profile, the hospital, and the practitioners. Health care in the United States is plentiful, but it is not distributed equally, nor is all health care of equal quality. One issue that these laws deal with is reduction of the inequities in both distribution and level of quality of health care. Another is controlling the cost of health care.

Because hospitals and other health-care agencies are a part of the larger health industry, the single organization is influenced by trends in the industry as a whole. Likewise, since each health-care agency is part of the broader industry, the sum total of the industry's effectiveness is determined to a large extent by the effectiveness of each agency. Quality assurance is an overall goal to control the industry, as well as a goal for control within each organizational entity. Quality assurance incorporates issues of accessibility to care, the effectiveness of care, and continuity of care, as well as cost containment. Practitioners who provide the care and consumers who receive it are the people who activate the system for quality assurance and who exercise control.

ACTIVATING THE PROCESS OF CONTROL

Controlling in an organization is multifaceted. For purposes of discussing organizational control, it is useful to think of control as a process that is activated by people. The process of control is activated by both practitioners and consumers who use material resources and who are influenced by environmental factors. Clinical effectiveness of patient care, the purpose of the health-care agency, depends on how people interact in admitting patients, providing care measures, teaching, referring, counseling, and ensuring the continuity of care. Quality care is often spoken of in idealistic terms, but the values assigned to these terms are sometimes different. Quality is actually demonstrated in the actions of the "controllers" of care, and these actions are determined by the different value systems of people. Family values, genetic traits, cultural and religious values are a few of the variables that influence decisions made by both the consumers and the practitioners who are involved in health care.

EXTERNAL SOURCES OF CONTROL

Organizations are dynamic and thus are changing continually in response to many factors, such as changes in society, changes in the technology of care, and new insights into the interpretation of health care. Today's issues in health care include how hospitals and other health-care agencies can change and adapt to increasing public demands and governmental regulation for quality and cost containment. Both have far-reaching implications in health-care organizations. These implications range from questioning the basic values of the health-care providers to changing specific methods used in organizations for such things as collecting data, keeping records, providing services, and generally accounting for the organization's activities. Hospitals and medical-care providers have not previously been accustomed to "outside" surveillance or to external controls to the extent being encountered at this time. Therefore, coping with external controls is becoming a predominant concern of administrators and health-care professionals.

To adapt to the increasing external control of health care, administrative and provider professionals are going through a stage of exploration and of learning how to cope with the demands for quality and for cost containment. Institutional practices are being questioned, as well as the value of certain care procedures and practices. In the processes of adapting and changing, professionals of all types who are involved in health-care agencies are learning and consequently developing new methods and new approaches for rendering health care in organizations.

ADAPTATION TO CHANGE IN ORGANIZATIONS
An article written by Argyris [1] provides some useful insights into the ongoing process of organizational learning and adaptation to change. Argyris describes organizational learning as a process of detecting and correcting error. He speaks of the tendency for norms to develop within organizations. In some organizations employees are afraid to "get into trouble" and consequently hide their errors so that a "network of camouflage and deception" develops. To counteract this, he suggests that a system for obtaining valid information be developed in which employees make a commitment to choice and to constant monitoring of implementation of the organization's work. To create this climate, he suggests that internal assumptions made within the organizations should be based on attitudes that power derives from having reliable information, from competence, from responsible employees, and from continual monitoring of the effects of decisions. Managers, to create this climate, develop a support system of advocacy for employees and establish relationships that both encourage inquiry and tolerate confrontation.

ENCOURAGING PARTICIPATION IN CONTROLLING
Controlling is often interpreted as use of power at the expense of other people. Argyris proposes that information is the source of power and controlling is a process through which people grow and develop by participating in decisions, by evaluating the effects of behaviors, and by taking corrective action. Argyris describes some of the dilemmas of people who have the power to control; these include the need to be a strong manager yet being open about the existence of dilemmas, being able to be open and yet not controlling, being an advocate and at the same time encouraging confrontation, being able to respond effectively to employees who are anxious even though the manager may also feel anxious, and finally being able to manage one's own fear and at the same time help people to overcome their fears.

These thoughts are pertinent to managers, particularly to those who are just beginning a career that entails management responsibilities. There are always problems and issues that managers must deal with. In the health-care system, solving these problems and issues involves not only the personnel who work within the organization, but also the consumer or recipient of health care. Providers of care are sometimes reluctant to solve these problems in groups that involve participation of consumers. They feel that the problems are professional ones and that involving consumers in their solution can hinder the trust that is basic to the consumer-professional relationship in health care. Consumers (patients) do, however, participate in health-care processes and can provide input that can be used to improve health care. Joint discussions of the health-care problems can be productive—consumers and practitioners often have common concerns about events.

The Role of Professionals in Controlling

Consumers of health care are participating increasingly in formal groups, such as committees or regulatory bodies that evaluate health-care quality and expenditures. But the consumers, while confronting issues of quality in health-care systems, still rely on the judgment of professionals in matters of professional knowledge and use of medical technology. The professional then has the prime responsibility in any quality assurance program or other type of controlling process in health care.

VALUE SYSTEM

Let us consider the role of the professional in controlling. The basis for control of any human effort is the value system of those who provide care and of those who use this care. Values influence what people consider to be important, necessary, or desirable when making choices. The choices that are made in organizations about what to control represent the values of the people, both consumers and professionals, who are making decisions. Consumers may participate in making these decisions, but they often rely on professional expertise to evaluate or to guide the direction of the decisions. It is an aspect of professionalism that the professionals will actively take the lead in controlling health care.

ETHICAL DECISION-MAKING

Basically, control processes begin with each professional. Organizational control is an aggregate of "professional control," and controlling in an organization is an interactive process that is subject to interpretations and to actions of people. The care choices made by practitioners are often ethical choices—determining whether an action is good or bad or right or wrong. Making choices is essentially decision-making. This ethical decision-making involves knowing the circumstances of a situation, knowing about one's freedom in making choices, evaluating and analyzing the alternative actions, determining the nature of the action (whether the person has a choice in the action), and judging the action according to principles or guidelines that will promote the most good.

The professional who is "in touch with his or her own reality" looks at care decisions as voluntary choices that have good and bad or right and wrong values. The health-care practitioner learns the principles or guidelines for making such judgments in a basic professional educational program and continues to update knowledge throughout the duration of practice. Values become clarified and firmed up through practice, and professionals become increasingly aware of their own values in making the difficult decisions about matters that arise in the course of a lifetime of practice.

SELF-CONTROL

Making decisions intentionally is an element of self-control. A system activated by human action is largely controlled by each person in the system. Control of the quality of health care—a broad endeavor—is accomplished in many ways, but the self-control exercised by knowledgeable workers who give health care is an important underlying element. Consistency in making decisions despite the pressures and stresses of daily events requires self-control. The consistency comes from inner sources—the person who is committed to a value system and who voluntarily makes decisions based on the values felt intuitively, as well as those known and expressed, can maintain consistency in behaviors. This consistency is viewed as control that is exercised when a person uses knowledge in making judgments that affect not only the person but also the person's use of resources and the behaviors the person exhibits when dealing with others in the care arena.

PROFESSIONAL SELF-REGULATION

Self-control is also applicable to a professional group. Self-regulation is an attribute of a profession. The regulation exercised by professionals within their group has ethical applications. A profession has a code of ethics that serves as a guide to professional judgment. Professionals provide a service that society requires and sanctions. They have a body of knowledge that is unique to the profession and that is applied in making judgments when providing the professional service, in accord with the code of ethics. Peer review is a technique used for professional self-regulation that reinforces self-control in individuals. The ability of a professional group to regulate its actions is an expectation of the society that sanctions the profession. This self-regulation is a basis for trust that individuals develop in their expectations of quality service provided by the professionals.

CONTROL BY AN AGGREGATE OF PROFESSIONALS

When several different professionals form an organization there is an aggregate of professional values. While the health-care professionals such as administrators, doctors, nurses, and others have a common interest in providing quality care, their functions may differ. The values inherent in these different functions may seem to conflict because each professional group has a different knowledge base and a different function, uses different terminology, and has a different perspective. Nurses, for example, approach patient care from the point of view of nurturing the patient in order to control illness or disease and maintain health. Doctors approach patient care from the perspective of diagnosis, treatment, and preventive measures. Administrators approach patient care from the perspective of using resources effectively and containing costs so that the organizational operations that support patient-care processes will be efficient.

DEVELOPMENT OF A COMMON TERMINOLOGY FOR CONTROL

Nurses may perceive conflict in values when their terminology for describing quality patient care does not harmonize with the terminology of budget management that is important to the administrator's function. Administrators take courses in finance, accounting, and systems management. Nurses take courses in nursing process and care of the patient. An ability to translate nursing process and patient care into fiscal management terms is a process of "enlightenment." Current emphasis on the development of quality assurance programs is providing a medium for professionals to work together to determine how their aggregate of functions can be blended for effectiveness and efficiency in patient care.

Nurses involved in quality control programs are learning how to phrase their idealistic sounding or broad terminology of patient-care goals in statements of standards that are becoming increasingly specific and consequently more adaptable to translation into the terminology of other health-related professional groups. One of the goals of quality assurance programs is to actualize a health-care delivery system that clearly delineates care values that can be related directly to efficiency values such as cost containment.

The Control Process

Professionals activate the control process. This process can be narrowly viewed as measuring outcomes. Examples of this approach are using predetermined standards to evaluate whether a cake is satisfactory after baking or whether a painting is satisfactory after the paint has dried. The process of control can also be viewed as measuring the means to achieve the outcomes as well as the final result. Traffic controls exemplify this approach. A speed limit is set as a standard of behavior: 20 mph in a school zone, 30 mph in normal city traffic, 55 mph on the highway. These speed limits represent a standard for safety in the designated category of area. In a school zone, 55 mph is an unsafe speed, and 20 mph is an unsafe speed for highway driving. The speed limits are the standards used to control the outcomes, in this illustration, public safety, which can be measured by the outcome goal of no traffic accidents.

Once the standard has been determined, there is an enforcer (a policeman) who measures vehicular speed. This person measures the speed of vehicles and compares the actual speed to the standard to reveal the differences, if any, between the vehicular speed and this standard. The enforcer controls by regulation—by stopping the noncomplying driver and giving a speeding ticket. The enforcer is implementing a plan of "corrective action." The principle of this corrective action is that knowledge of the regulation is well known by drivers, since to be licensed they must pass an examination that tests their knowledge of traffic laws. The driver also knows what the consequences of failure to comply will be. The speeding ticket is designed to make an impact on the person who does not comply—it serves as a force for behavioral modification so that the driver will comply with the standard in the future. If the driver repeatedly fails to comply, there are further corrective actions that can be used, such as loss of license or mandatory participation in driving classes.

CONTROL BY THE HEALTH-CARE PROFESSIONAL

The manager applies the components of the control process to the patient-care situation. Although speed limits are more easily translated into standards than are nursing-care measures, the same components apply. In nursing, both the methods used in giving patient care and the outcomes are important for the patient's safety and welfare. The processes of care or events that take place throughout the patient's health-care experience can be delineated and can be controlled. The outcomes of care can also be defined and controlled.

Measuring quality care is a complex matter. Consider the patient-care process from your nursing perspective. There are certain aspects of care that are confined to the discrete relationship between the nurse and the patient. You and the patient could interact to implement these aspects of care in any setting: in the patient's home, in the hospital, or in a waiting room or conference room. Such nursing process components that are interactive in nature are teaching, counseling, emotional support, and history taking for assessment. Other aspects of the patient-care process require materials, supplies, and a controlled environment. Surgery, for example, is conducted in an aseptic environment and requires sterile equipment, specialized operating room equipment, monitoring devices, and sterile supplies. In order to assure quality patient care in these types of situations, not only the care processes, but also the environmental and operational processes that support care must be measured. The care processes include not only nursing functions, but also the specialized professional functions of others.

CONTROL BY THE PATIENT
In addition to the control exercised by people in the organization, patients can also exercise control in the health-care system. Patient's behaviors are often measured in quality assurance programs. Because the patient does not have to comply with care measures and is not a part of the organization, controversy can arise about whether these behaviors are actually a measurement of the quality of care given. Consider, for example, that people have a right to health care. Such rights or interests are provided for by law, and health-care providers have a duty to respect and provide these rights. A right implies, however, that an individual may choose to exercise the right or not, according to personal wishes. Providers have a duty to provide care, but patients have the right to accept or not to accept care. A provider may, for example, prescribe the correct medication for a patient's condition, but the patient does not have to purchase or take this medication. This explanation is an oversimplification of rights and duties, but it serves to describe the relationship between a health-care practitioner and a patient.

It is important that the practitioners perceive patients' rights for health care as interests that the patient controls. A patient does not have to comply with health care. When a given patient exercises this right to noncompliance, he or she is making a value judgment. As with professionals, the patients' values are the basis for their decisions about how they will participate in the health care. The professionals may provide all the necessary care processes and operational requisites for quality care, but the patient influences the outcomes by choosing how or whether to comply with treatment measures. To measure the outcomes of care in terms of patient's compliance with care is complex because noncompliance does not always imply that the health-care practitioners did not give "quality care." On the other hand, one of the professional duties is to develop methods through which patients can learn how to comply with their health-care measures on the basis of understanding the importance of the care for their ongoing health.

Quality Assurance Programs

Quality assurance programs conducted by nurses involve a process of self-regulation that demonstrates how nursing behaviors affect patient progress. These programs are related to the entire spectrum of quality assurance activities being conducted within the health-care industry. In this industry there are several factors that are considered in determining the quality of care. These include accessibility to care (which can be limited by distance, lack of transportation, limited hours, inability to pay, organizational barriers that cause delays in appointments or admissions, and obstructive behaviors by health-care personnel) and the beliefs and attitudes of patients about their health care. These factors tend to be measured by evaluating the patient's delay in obtaining and receiving care, the patient's failure to follow up with prescribed care, and the health-delivery system's use by people in a geographic location.

Another dimension of quality assurance is the structure of health care. This is defined as the organizational structure of health-care agencies, methods of financing care, and personnel staffing of the organizations. The process of care is yet another dimension and is defined as the professional-patient contact. Professional competence, which includes both technical and interpersonal skills of the health-care providers, is a common factor used to measure the process of care. Outcomes of care represent another dimension of quality assurance. These outcomes include the patient's ability to function as a result of health care and the patient's satisfaction with the health care. Outcomes can also be measured by evaluating the health status of a population.

Professional nurses are concerned with self-regulation within this health-care system. An important point made by Davidson in a non-health care related article applies to nurses. He states that "professions devote themselves to public needs defined by the public but also have developed their own institutions for serving needs defined by their own parochial conception of the public interest" [3].

Quality assurance programs are concerned then not only with professional behaviors and with structural dimensions of the health-care system, but also with the patients' expectations of health care. One of the complex issues in quality assurance programs is defining the relationships between professional standards of care and the patients' expectations of care. Evaluation of quality must also include determining the relationships among the structure, the process, and the outcome dimensions of health-care delivery. Information about these relationships is important to determine how to improve the system. Thus far, research efforts have not revealed any clear relationships among structure, process, and outcomes [4].

UTILIZATION REVIEWS

One way of evaluating care is through the utilization reviews required by Medicare and Medicaid. The utilization reviews include appropriateness of the patient's admission to the hospital, the patient's length of stay, and the number of services used in the care of the patient. Utilization reviews can be conducted concurrently with the patient's hospital stay or can be done retrospectively by evaluating the medical records following the patient's discharge.

AUDITS

An audit is another commonly used measure to determine the effectiveness of care. The audit consists of developing a plan in which pertinent questions are answered: (1) What is the standard of quality to be achieved? (2) Why should the standard be achieved? (3) Where, when, by whom, and how should the standard be implemented in the health-care system?

Design of the audit procedure and forms used for auditing are based on the answers to these questions. The design of the audit program specifies what is to be tested in the audit, the standard for measurement, comparison of what actually happened with this standard, and evaluation of the degree of conformity that has been achieved in attempts to meet the standard. The time frame for conducting the audit is also part of the design and can include all of the activities that take place from the time that the patient is admitted to the hospital to the time of the patient's discharge.

Assessment of the patient's status at the time of admission provides the data used to determine the baseline for evaluating changes that take place during the hospitalization. (Certificate of need required by PSRO legislation is designed to document the patient's status at the time of admission.) Once the patient is admitted, the processes of care are evaluated to determine what nursing actions took place. The end result of the patient's care is measured by the assessment completed at the time of the patient's discharge. Evaluation of this flow of care can be the basis for interpreting the effects of the hospitalization, but this interpretation must take into account factors that were not controllable by the patient, the professionals, or the structure.

An audit is most effective if it is related to the overall goals of the nursing department in the health-care agency. To conduct such an audit voluntarily is indicative of professional accountability and represents how organizations can learn, as described earlier. Audits can be designed to measure any number of aspects of patient care; those aspects selected for audit represent the value system as defined in the nursing organization's goals. One effect of audits is that they bring attention to the aspects of care being measured. It is important to develop measures that assess both what nurses consider to be important in patient care and what patients consider to be important in order to gain the most relevant feedback that can be used to improve care.

Professional groups have different perspectives about the importance of different aspects of patient care. Greene [4] cites that the dimensions of priorities for quality assurance vary for government, consumers, and professionals. He states that governmental priorities are efficiency and effectiveness. Consumer priorities are accessibility and acceptability. Professional priorities are provider competence and effectiveness. Greene states that there is overlap among these dimensions. A long-range goal to be achieved is to determine whether all of these priorities can be related to one another in developing methods to improve the quality of health care. The current state of the art is early-stage development of measures of quality. Because audits are often used to measure the quality of nursing care, we shall examine the audit procedure.

THE AUDIT PROCEDURE

An audit is application of the control process. The basis for an audit is determination of the standard of care. This standard is written prior to conducting the audit and is stated specifically so that it can be measured against actual practice. Conducting an audit requires a decision about "what" is to be measured. This means that the standard of care should be written with criteria similar to the speed limit example. One of the concerns of the auditor is making choices about which standards to measure that will "test" or compare what actually happened with what should have happened. Following the measurement or test, there is the need for corrective action if discrepancies have been found. This corrective action is the mechanism through which future events are controlled for quality.

To be meaningful, the standards of care selected for audit have to be an index of quality. What standards are measurable? By what criteria? How do these standards measure quality? Patient care is complex and, if comprehensive and holistic, is difficult to measure. How do you know if a patient's emotional needs for preoperative support were adequately met? How do you know if counseling sessions for a patient achieved any results? How do you know if your teaching of a patient was effective? Which standards of care can you select for measurement to gain adequate information about the quality of care given?

In many instances, standards of care are determined by groups of nurses who are giving care. The group determination of standards is a developmental process that uses the concept of the value of group participation. The value of the use of groups as the vehicle for determining standards of care is that a consensus can be reached about what standards ought to be. Nurses who participate in determining what standards ought to be apply their cognitive knowledge of nursing to statements of criteria about what events determine quality in the care process. Awareness of the importance of these events serves to help nurses translate the words into actions when giving care. This developmental process is an exercise that in itself is a control device that heightens the practitioner's awareness of assessment factors, procedures, techniques, and methods of care. This heightened awareness colors the nurse's actions since it focuses the nurse's attention on these standards when giving care.

Written Standards. Written standards of care are valuable in the control process. These written standards are a consistent and retrievable data base for "testing" care actually given. They are also a reference for nurses who are giving care. Such references enable the nurse to "stabilize" care processes. When one considers the vast amount of knowledge applicable to patient care, the numerous interruptions the nurse is subject to in the course of a day, and the great demand to relate to patients and personnel at all levels of communication, references are invaluable in stabilizing the direction of actions. Nurses "think on their feet," but they are human, and when overloaded with sensory input, they cannot always think of all the important aspects of care for every patient without assisting devices.

Another purpose of written standards is that they serve to inform nurses (employees) of the expectations of their work. Knowledge of what is expected in performance and feedback about the effects of performance are important in motivation. When performance is visibly related to a tangible measurement, one can obtain feedback necessary for continued motivation. The process of developing and writing standards clarifies the expectations of the nurse in the employment setting; it also clarifies the role of the nurse for others.

The process of determining and writing standards has another advantage—those who participate in the process broaden their perspectives of care. A standard has to have a basis in fact, in theory, or in some background information that substantiates and validates the standard. To investigate an area of care implies that the committee or group classifies, categorizes, and conceptualizes and then derives tangible criteria from the data. What is generally present or true, what happens in most cases, and what determines whether this care process is effective for patients with this classification of illness or disease are questions that committee members must answer.

Relationships among events become more clear when writing standards. Consider the following example:

If a patient has _____, the patient will experience emotional and physiological responses of _____ that require _____ intervention. The patient is subject to _____ complications and can be expected to progress toward wellness or advance through the phases of _____. The patient requires _____ information or assistance to regain or retain maximum health consisting of _____.

Filling in the blanks directs attention to developing normative expectations of care for patients with certain categories of problems. By viewing these patients in a classification or category, one's perspective is generalized and therefore broadened.

Determining Realistic Standards. Where do the data for these generalizations come from? Some sources include information from books and other media about pathophysiology; about treatment and therapies to determine what interventions restore, correct, or supplement the disrupted physiological mechanisms; about patients' responses to determine the normal course of events when certain physiologic or emotional disturbances occur; and about the complications that can occur as a result of the original disturbance, the treatment or therapies, or patients' responses to them. Standards based on theory and on observations of actual practice are more likely to be realistic and possible to achieve; these are both important factors in measuring such standards. The ANA standards of care can also be used as professional normative guidelines for developing standards.

Why should standards be realistic and possible to achieve? The importance of realism in standard setting has many implications. From a performance point of view, the standards or expectations must be attainable. Being expected to carry out performance standards that are beyond the ordinary capabilities of practitioners is frustrating. With such high standards, the practitioner could well react with the attitude, Why try since it's impossible? To engender motivation to perform well, standards must be perceived as attainable.

Another reason why standards should be attainable is that they must be accepted by practitioners if they are to become part of that person's repertory. The person makes a commitment to achieve standards, and this commitment implies agreement with and capability for carrying out the standard. People need to be successful in carrying out commitments to fulfill their own feelings of need satisfaction. A self-actualizing person has needs to achieve, and these needs are thwarted when the standards are not realistic or if only "supernurse" could attain them.

Written standards not only commit the practitioners to a level of performance, but they also commit the organization to that level of performance. A written standard can potentially be used in a legal action if a patient brings suit. The same test used in audits of comparing the standard to the actual events is used to determine "what should have happened" in legal actions. The standard then becomes a "duty" that the nurse has to patients. One way of managing this use of standards is to clarify in writing that they are guidelines for practice or goals to be developed through continued assessment and improvement. Standards are not actually normative in nature until they are studied over a period of time and data from the studies are measured statistically on the basis of actual performance to find "normative" ranges of practice. It should also be mentioned that the written standard of care cannot be applied equally to all patients' care because of the variability among patients in their motivations for care and for cure, their responses to treatment, and other intervening variables. The normative standard that applies to a patient's condition is always subject to change according to the patient's condition and progress.

Conducting an Audit. The process of implementing an audit has both developmental and organizational implications. It is developmental in that the people who conduct the audit and those whose actions are being audited can learn from the feedback derived from the audit. It has organizational implications since the audit may reveal deficiencies in policies, procedures, rules, or methods of operations used to support patient care. The use of feedback from the audit, if validity in measures is ensured, is an impetus to evaluating the total patient-care situation. Audits are, however, made on the basis of chart documentation and have the potential for measuring expertise in charting rather than what actually happened in the care process.

It is important that everyone who participates in the audit process be informed about the procedures being used so that input and learning can be a part of the process from the outset. The audit is a procedure that is conducted by specified people, but it measures the effects of nursing actions in general and every attempt should be made to ensure that the feedback gleaned from auditing will be relevant. The audit itself is conducted according to specified conditions. An audit is a controlled evaluation. It is controlled, just as a scientific experiment is controlled, to ensure that measurement will be reliable and valid.

There are several approaches to conducting an audit. The method of the Joint Commission for Accreditation of Hospitals uses criteria for outcomes, 24 hours prior to discharge. Patients' charts are reviewed according to these outcome criteria but in retrospect, that is, after the patient is discharged. The review criteria are stated in terms of expected outcomes that should have occurred 24 hours prior to discharge. Complications are indications that these expected outcomes were not met. If complications have occurred, the chart is examined to isolate factors that may have influenced development of the complications. Assessment, treatment, therapy, and other process factors are evaluated to determine if care was given according to process standards for prevention of the complications. This evaluation indicates whether the complications could have been prevented and whether they were detected and managed appropriately. Decisions are then made about the data so that remedial action can be taken.

Another commonly used system is the Medicus System. This system uses both process and outcome criteria. The criteria used include admission data, events that took place during hospitalization called interim data, and outcome data taken at the time of discharge.

Selection of charts for audit is usually based on the most frequently occurring category of patients. Not every patient chart is audited. Instead a representative sample is selected to evaluate care during a stated time frame—one month, three months, six months. Factors that influence the audit include the number of patient-care units represented, the staff turnover, and the number of patients within a given category. Patient charts are selected according to diagnosis, the reason for hospitalization, or other criteria selected for standards in the audit. Often patients have multiple health problems, but the diagnosis for the current hospitalization is the "primary diagnosis" used for an audit of events during this time period. In the patient charts the auditors check the nursing notes, the progress notes, measurement graphs for TPR or blood pressure, and medication chart forms. A summary of the audit results is distributed according to procedure, and the results are coded to protect the unit or staff identity, to maintain objectivity. The data are retrievable, however, to isolate factors that have contributed to the care.

A summary report of the audit includes the category of patient audited, the time of the patients' admission and discharge, the number of patient charts reviewed, the reason for the sample selection method, the age and sex of the patients, the number of patient-care units included, and the names of the auditors. The findings of the test for criteria, the data collected for each criterion, the percentage index of compliance, and other data that might be included are recorded by patient-care area. These findings are used as feedback to analyze the reasons for noncompliance present at the time the patients were in the hospital.

Analysis of Audit Results. The process of evaluation begins with analyzing the audit findings. If noncompliance in a given area is demonstrated, the reasons for noncompliance are investigated. Possible reasons are multiple. One may be that charting documentation was inadequate, another that staff turnover temporarily influenced the quality of care. Other reasons may include a large number of new orientees, problems related to use of equipment or supplies, environmental deficits, problems in communication networks, deficits in nursing knowledge, or inadequate staffing. The documentation of problems is the basis for corrective action. To be pertinent and relevant, corrective action must be directly related to the "root" problems identified. The type and duration of corrective action are based on the nature of the problem, and usually the solution is not as simple as giving a traffic ticket. Staff development activities, for example, may require a course or a series of workshops to remedy problems. Revision of the charting system may be another remedy, as are such activities as establishing better communication networks, improving charting, or working with other hospital personnel to improve delivery of supplies.

The analysis of audit results is usually conducted by a committee. This committee examines the results to interpret their meaning. Situational factors mentioned earlier, such as professional to non-professional nursing staff ratios, are explored in relation to the audit results. Review of situational factors is important in determining the causes of deficiencies or discrepancies. Interpretation of the data is basic to developing plans for corrective action.

Use of audit committees to interpret data is practiced in industries other than the health-care industry. Lovdal [5] studied thirteen New York Stock Exchange companies and found that the most effective results of audits were the results of deliberations of audit committees. Some of the practices he cites that were found to augment the effectiveness of audit committees are balanced membership of the committee, a flow of complete information to the committee, independence from the executive officer, and periodic self-assessment of the committee.

The purpose of an audit committee is to review the data in terms of changes in current practice that could be made to improve care. The data must be evaluated according to situational factors to prevent errors in interpretation. It is also important that the audit committee base the interpretations on fact, principles, and theories as much as possible to prevent inappropriate judgments. Many factors can create dissonance in interpretation of audit data among individuals; changes in norms of the standards of care, new rules and regulations relating to federal and state laws, new technology, organizational practices, and changes within the health-care delivery system in a community can all influence interpretation of data.

Corrective action taken on the basis of audit data, if viewed in the broader perspective of the organization, has many implications. Interpretation of audit data can be the impetus for change in nursing-care practices that in turn can have impact on the organizational operations or on relationships among people in the organization. The overall goal is to improve patient care. Improvements suggested must be rational and cost-effective if they are to be implemented.

Qualitative Versus Quantitative Data

Quality assurance programs are designed to measure "qualitative" data. This is an effort that not only is difficult to define with any degree of universally accepted specificity, but that also taxes the imagination and the creativity of the evaluators. These programs are expensive, and some types of measurements, such as audits, are more expensive than others. The effort of measuring quality is useful and worth the expenditure only if it results in improved patient care.

Qualitative data are nominal and difficult to standardize, while quantitative data are much more amenable to measurement since they involve collecting information about tangible and visible aspects of care. Qualitative data are concerned with factors such as the effects of treatment and medication measures evaluated by the progress in the patient's cure. Quantitative data measure factors such as how much of what kind of medication was used, how many dressing packs were used, and how much nursing time was spent with the patient performing care activities. Nurses are becoming increasingly sophisticated in their knowledge of the importance of both qualitative and quantitative data. The remainder of this chapter will explore some of the issues and methods used by nurses to use quantitative data in control of patient care.

The Budget

A budget is a plan of how an organization will allocate its money resources in a given period of time for the purchase of other resources necessary to function. The processes of planning budgets and of quality assurance programs are similar in that both are based on value judgments about health care. In quality assurance programs the judgments are made in planning standards of care to be measured. In budgetary planning, the value judgments are made in planning how to allocate institutional resources according to the health-care services that are needed or desired. Both budgets and quality assurance programs are concerned with efficiency and equality in health-care services, but they approach these concerns from different perspectives.

EQUATING QUALITY WITH COST

Quality assurance programs attempt to identify the effectiveness of health care from the perspective of qualitative standards. These qualitative standards sometimes are not easily applied to specific tangibles such as costs for manpower or the amount of space or supplies required for quality care. The budget is an attempt to identify how limited organizational resources can be allocated throughout the organization to provide the most effective health care. The specific and tangible resources such as cost of manpower, space, and supplies are equated with standards of care offered through health-care services in the organization. The issue of how to translate qualitative standards into quantitative measures of cost is central in both budgetary planning and in quality assurance programs. The different perspectives in approach for each of these control processes make them seem dichotomous or even incongruent. It is perhaps an oversimplification to state that the two different types of control measures have the same end goal because the perspectives of each differ. Grave questions such as, Can we assign a dollar value to human life? or on the other hand, Can we determine what level of quality in health care is affordable given limited dollar resources? are underlying the issues of effectiveness and equality in health care.

PHILOSOPHY OF BUDGETING

This introduction to budgets is designed to help you consider budgetary planning in the broad perspective of total organizational planning. Philosophies and values may seem tangential when you are actually planning a budget because numbers don't look like concepts such as quality or human life values. It is useful to think of budgets in terms of philosophy and values to overcome the constraining aspects of budgeting and to emphasize the strategical aspects of the budget process. In this process of budgeting, one considers how to get the best value from limited dollar resources. The idea of best value for dollars spent is one you probably deal with every day in decisions you make. If you are hungry, for example, and you have a quarter to spend for food, should you buy an orange or a package of cookies? This decision requires knowledge of available choices and is made on the basis of value judgments, your feelings, attitudes, and habits, as well as knowledge of the nutritional value of foods and body needs for nutrients.

BUDGETING LIMITED RESOURCES

You can identify with the concept of limited dollar resources in your own life. You earn a specific amount of money from which you determine your expenditures. You are limited in your purchases of goods and services by the amount of your income. An organization, such as a health-care agency, also has to function within the limitations imposed by resources available. Money is one of these resources, and money is used by the organization to purchase other necessary resources. Decisions have to be made about how to allocate the money available to the agency for these other resources: people, supplies, and equipment. These decisions are crucial in determining the scope of patient-care services that the agency will provide.

A Budget as a Future Plan. The purpose of a budget is to make rational decisions about how much money you need and about how you will spend your money. In formulating a plan for income and expenditures, you think of your goals for the budget period just as an organization plans a budget according to goals. Because the immediate and long-range future is full of unknowns, the organization forecasts future events in the budget period just as you try to think of all the upcoming expenditures that you must meet or that you will desire to make in the future.

A Budget as a Control Device. A budget is a control device because it allocates expenditures and this allocation serves as a "standard" for the actual expenditures that are made throughout the budget period. When more money is spent than was allocated for certain items, corrective action is taken. This corrective action is based on evaluation of the reasons why the budgetary standard was not followed. Reasons might include finding that unnecessary expenditures were made, that the projected costs of items was unrealistic or that costs had increased after the budget was planned, or that not all costs for a given activity were planned for in the initial budget.

In planning a budget, it is necessary to project costs as accurately as possible. The allocation of expenditures in an organization is made according to some type of framework, and there is usually a format or guide for making out the budget that is followed by all persons involved in budgetary planning throughout the institution. Budgets for organizations are usually separated according to departments, programs, or special projects.

ALLOCATION OF ORGANIZATIONAL RESOURCES
The manager who is planning the budget for a specific department or unit within a department follows the organizational format for planning. When all departmental program or project budgets have been completed, the entire organizational budget can be prepared. Using a common format enables the central budget committee to prepare the master organizational budget more easily since a consistent approach has been made by all planners. After developing the entire organizational budget from the separate budgets, it may be necessary to decrease amounts in certain areas to comply with total organizational dollar resources. Budgets submitted by people from various departments are approved following total organizational review and revision of projected income and expenditures.

Types of Costs Included in Budgets. Budgets usually include different types of costs: those that occur consistently, those that vary, and major expenditures for equipment or for building projects. The consistent costs, called fixed costs, include items such as plant maintenance, salaries, supplies, and equipment rentals that are made on an annual basis. Fixed costs remain stable despite the amount of use or volume of services. Costs that change with the amount of use or volume of services are called variable costs. An example of a variable cost for a patient-care unit is supplies such as dressings or pharmaceuticals that are used as patients require. If the census of the patient-care unit includes 15 patients who require dressing changes in one week and only 5 patients who require dressing changes in another, costs for supplies will vary, being greater when there are 15 patients using them than when there are only 5.

Capital Expenditures. Major expenditures for equipment are capital expenditures. These capital costs include purchases of equipment that is expensive but that is expected to be used for many years. The capital equipment costs are figured over a lifetime of expected service. An x-ray machine, an examining table, or an auto-analyzer are examples of capital expenditures. Equipment that is less costly is called minor equipment and includes such items as small tape recorders and sphygmomanometers. Minor equipment items may be included in operating costs or in equipment costs.

Operating Costs. Operating costs are those expenditures necessary for maintaining the ongoing services or day-to-day functions throughout the budget period. Operating costs are "what it costs to operate the service unit." These costs differ from capital expenditures in that the capital expenditures are made for items that maintain value during the item's lifetime. An automobile, for example, is a capital expenditure that you might make. It has a continuing value that depreciates over time. The items required to maintain the function of your car, such as gasoline, oil, and antifreeze, are operating costs. If you always drive your car the same number of miles each day, these operating costs are consistent or "fixed." If you drive your car a different number of miles each day, the operating costs are variable and depend on the amount of use. The license plates and insurance for your car are fixed costs.

DATA BASED BUDGET PROJECTIONS
You can estimate the costs for your automobile from your past experiences. Your previous bills for gas, oil, and other maintenance costs provide you with data to use in projecting future costs. Data are also the basis for forecasting organizational budgets. These data are obtained from review of past costs, from comparison of costs throughout the organization, and from evaluating methods of operations that have taken place in the past. Data must be analyzed to determine whether there might be a better and more efficient way to operate. It is not sufficient to say that past costs are an indication of future needs. Data can also be used to evaluate real costs over a period of time to determine which costs have remained stable and which costs have changed or fluctuated. The reasons for fluctuations can then be evaluated to determine the internal or external factors that influence costs.

Analysis of Data. Analyzing data to determine factors that influence costs is used in budgeting to develop strategy. The effects of changes in patient census, the mix of patients according to acuity of illness or diagnostic categories, the mix of staff (RN, LPN, or NA), the methods used to accomplish work, and the types of services rendered are some of the major areas that can be analyzed to develop strategies for spending organizational dollars more effectively. Strategic aspects of budgeting are most challenging. Developing strategies for budgeting includes not only evaluation of material resources but also the potential of employees for functioning. Because health-care agencies are generally labor intensive, the function of employees is the central focus of many strategic plans.

EVALUATING THE COSTS AND BENEFITS OF RESOURCES
There are several ways to approach an evaluation of the potential of employees for functioning when developing strategies for budgeting. One approach is to evaluate what types of material resources the employees need to carry out their functions. A nurse who is carrying out teaching plans for patients with chronic illness needs printed materials and other forms of media as teaching-learning resources. Administering medications requires medicine cups, syringes, medicine carts, chart forms, requisition slips, inventories of medications, and other such material resources. In budgeting, expenses are planned according to the materials and people necessary to fulfill the roles specified by the operational activity. The benefits of the activity must justify the cost.

Manpower Resources. Another approach to developing budgetary strategy is to evaluate the capabilities of employees. The use of material resources requires decision-making by employees. The types of decisions made may require special educational preparation or particular talents. A registered nurse, by virtue of education, can make decisions about the use of resources in giving patient care that a licensed practical nurse would not be expected to make. The licensed practical nurse, in turn, makes decisions not expected of a nurse's aide. In addition to educational preparation, the unique talents and the experience of employees also contribute to their capability for management of resources. The capability to use resources effectively is one of the criteria that are considered in promotion of employees to management positions.

Mode of Operation. Another approach to developing budgetary strategies is to analyze the mode of operation used to accomplish work. Often more effective and economical ways of operation can be determined. To introduce changes in the way that people function together in an organization, whether the change involves use of a new technology, new equipment, or a new method of procurement of supplies, involves orientation or educational programs. Therefore, when making such changes it is necessary to forecast the types of problems that the employees may have in making the changes. The type of change being made may involve a role change for certain employees, or it may involve adapting to a new method for communicating with people in another department. If the change involves a redefinition of roles or functions, an educational program and development of support systems to help people adapt to the change must be included in the cost of the change.

Costs of Change. Costs that might be incurred in making operational changes are numerous. These costs may include rewriting and printing new procedure manuals; holding orientation meetings to introduce the employees to the new methods; writing, printing, and disseminating materials to employees to explain the new procedures and the reasons for their implementation; training sessions to learn about a new and sometimes complex technology; or continuing education programs or travel to other institutions to learn about different methods for accomplishing some particular function or to teach people about the conceptual rationale for changing. Continuing education costs may also be required to teach new content about a given area of professional practice that is required to implement the change in methods of operation. The capacities of the personnel and their needs for both training and development are integral parts of strategies developed in budgetary planning.

LONG-TERM EFFECTS OF A BUDGET

Many of the strategies developed in the budget process have long-term effects even though a budget is usually planned from year to year. Both the immediate future, which is the next year's budget that is being developed, and the long-range future are considered in developing any budget. Some programs may be expensive to initiate, but their costs are often figured over the long term if the change will effect savings over the long run. Going through the process of developing a budget for the coming year helps the personnel plan organizational activities and modes of operation in terms of what must be done to accommodate to changes in the organization, in professional fields, and in the expectations of the people who use the health-care services. These changes are ongoing, and an organization such as a hospital has to speculate about the future when planning strategies for the present. You can understand, therefore, that a budget has far-reaching effects in an organization.

COMMITMENT TO FUTURE ORGANIZATIONAL GOALS

The understanding that the future of the organization is considered in the present budgeting process is important. A budget is often perceived as a constraining force by personnel, and in a way it is. Making commitments to a plan of action in the budgeting process involves planning for allocation of resources in the future. The processes of "budgeting now" to accommodate future changes determine a direction that the organization will take in the programs and services offered. For this reason, it is difficult to make changes that are not included in the budgetary planning because any change may also change the direction of goals to be achieved and may require a different set of income and expenditure figures. The master budget may be planned so that changes are difficult to make unless there is an even exchange of costs, income, and benefits for one type of activity for another, or unless the new activity will earn as much as it costs. As a professional employee of an organization, you should consider your function in terms of the future and provide input for the budgeting process so that changes you perceive to be necessary can be considered at the time of budgeting.

TYPES OF BUDGETARY PLANS

Budgets are plans that assign dollar values to programs and services of the institution. There are several different ways to go about planning for the budget. *Incremental budgeting* is a method in which the previous year's budget is used as the basis for developing the new budget. *Zero-based budgeting* is a type of planning that emphasizes evaluation of programs and services in terms of the mission of the institution. In this process the specific department or budget area must justify its purposes. The planners prepare a description of the functions and intended purposes of the activities and then assign costs to these functions. A number of different ways for accomplishing these functions are planned, with costs for personnel, materials, and space determined for each of the plans. The costs and benefits of each plan are compared to finalize the area budget.

A *program budget* is similar to zero-based budgeting in that the costs of the program are evaluated in terms of its intended purposes. All of the costs that will be incurred in implementation of the program are evaluated in terms of the program goals. In program and in zero-based budgeting the master organizational budget is planned by evaluating the importance of each activity in view of the organization's goals. Priorities are made according to value systems, data available about patients' expectations of services, projected needs for services in the long run, professional standards, and the type of income or other benefit to the organization.

Budgets are often prepared according to line items. In the *line item budget* income and expenses are categorized into classes; this provides for data about specific types of costs. Differentiation of items enables the planner to forecast all the different types of expenditures that will be incurred and then to evaluate actual expenditures according to type. The line item budget is particularly useful if the different types of costs are appropriately defined for a given activity. When the budget in any line item is exceeded during the budget year, the reason for the overage can be pinpointed. If, for example, the budget for the line item maintenance of equipment is exceeded, one can immediately begin to evaluate why the equipment maintenance costs increased.

THE BUDGET AS AN EVALUATION TOOL

This brief description of the line item budget is included to demonstrate how a budget can be used to evaluate activities. As a manager, you are responsible for efficient and economical use of resources. If your expenditures in any one area, such as maintenance, exceed the amount planned for in the budget, you must investigate the cause. You may find that the equipment is old and cannot withstand wear. In this event, you would include purchase of new equipment to replace the worn-out equipment in the following year's capital budget. You might find that the personnel using the equipment do not know how to use it correctly. In this event, you would develop a plan for orientation or teaching to rectify misuse. Your evaluation might indicate that the equipment was recently used more frequently because a specific type of patient need had increased or because personnel were employed who use the equipment more frequently than past employees. In this case, your evaluation of the equipment involves analyzing the types of services that require its use. This evaluation may lead you to determine that the activities involved might be conducted in another way. You might find that the procedures or functions could be carried out more effectively and economically through different processes or by using a different type of equipment. In this event you would not simply replace the existing equipment with a similar type, but would redesign the function.

The Budget as a Source of Information. As with any control device, analysis of the budget provides information that is used as the basis for evaluation of activities in an organization. Spending more or less money than was allocated indicates that the manager needs to evaluate the differences by isolating problems that are being encountered. Likewise, when income differs from the amount projected, the services producing the income must be evaluated. The manager uses the budget as a source of information for future planning. The budget is a useful tool that helps the manager understand the effects of people, the workplace, and resources on each other. When used as a tool for management, the budget is not constraining, but serves as a guide and as a reminder of plans made for functions throughout the budget period.

THE BUDGET AS A TOOL FOR COMMUNICATION

A manager can learn to use budgets for many purposes. The purposes of budgets in planning have been described. It should be emphasized that budgets are one type of plan that is recognized as important by everyone in the organization. Budgets provide a common language for communicating with people in different professional groups and can be used as a medium of communication by the nurse-manager. Because budgets are common to the entire organization, planning the budget for a specific department and having this departmental plan reviewed by the budget committee that plans the organization's master budget serve to communicate programs and purposes. In many respects, acceptance of a departmental budget by a master planning committee implies acceptance of the department's purposes and goals by the organizational hierarchy.

The Budget as a Goal. Budgets are total organizational plans that quantify the organization's purposes and goals. Personnel in each department or program manage a part of the total organizational budget, and through this management fulfill broad organizational purposes. The budget then provides a direction for operation for all persons in the organization. It is theorized that when people in various departments are actively involved in the processes of budgetary planning, these people make a commitment to achieving the goals set forth in the budget. When this is the case, the process of budgetary planning and evaluation can be a source of motivation for employees.

The Budget as a Tool for Organizational Coordination. Analysis of budgets provides data that are used to evaluate the organization's activities. The data gleaned from budgets are useful not only to managers in specific departments but also to those who manage the entire organization. Budgetary processes, then, provide for coordination of activities within an organization. If maintenance costs have increased throughout the organization, for example, the spectrum of activities that take place in the organization and the types of external services purchased for maintenance are evaluated. This evaluation may lead to a change in plans made for the maintenance of equipment. Just as people in a specific department can evaluate their functions according to budgetary data, the administrators of the organization can evaluate activities in the entire organization from budgetary data.

THE BUDGET AS A TOTAL ORGANIZATIONAL PLAN

It is important, therefore, to consider that a budget is a plan for use of the organization's total resources. Everyone who is employed by the organization is accounted for in the budget through the inclusion of salaries and fringe benefits. In addition to these personnel costs, everyone who is employed uses the space and materials in the organization. Efficient and economical use by employees of all supplies, space, and equipment is necessary to control expenditures. Very small items, such as pens and paper products, can be large expenditures in the overall budget. Being careful in the use of material supplies is similar to saving pennies. Have you ever collected pennies in a jar for one month? And were you surprised to find how much money you had saved in just one month's time? As a manager, you are responsible for "saving pennies" in the way that you work with other people and in the way that you expect them to use materials and resources. You can better control costs in the area of your management responsiblity when you make every person fiscally responsible.

The Role of Nurses in Cost Containment

Nurses constitute the largest percentage of hospital employees. The productivity of nurses in providing patient-care services is therefore important in cost containment. Measurements of nursing productivity are not well defined. While a physician who sees patients in an office charges them for services rendered, nurses employed by hospitals are usually not paid directly by patients, nor are patients usually charged for specific nursing services. Nursing care has not previously been considered a cost center on the basis of services rendered in most hospitals. (A cost center is one in which separate accounting is made for a specific type of cost.)

DIFFERENTIATED NURSING-CARE COSTS

Stevens [6] and Bauer [2] suggest that nurses should determine methods for charging patients according to nursing-care needs. Stevens proposes that patients should be billed according to the level of care received, based on a patient classification system. If costs for nursing-care measures were specified, patients could be given information about the price of different services and could choose to use the services they are willing to pay for. Bauer proposes a nursing-care price index to measure and evaluate the costs of nursing services. By using a nursing-care price index, changes in costs could be more accurately measured in a given organization. A standard formula for a nursing-care price index could also be used to compare nursing-service costs in organizations that differ in size.

MEASURING NURSING PRODUCTIVITY

As a manager you are evaluated by your productivity, and you also evaluate other personnel according to their productivity. To measure productivity, one often relies on intuition and on evaluation of general performance. The nurse who is well organized, who is competent, who uses resources well, and who can complete care effectively and in sufficient quantity is generally termed "productive."

Nursing productivity is not easily defined in budgetary terms. To explore some of the facets of productivity one must consider the capabilities of the individual professional nurse, the organizational behaviors that have an impact on the nurse's function, the standards of nursing care on which evaluation of accomplishments is measured, and environmental factors that influence the nurse's practice. How the nurse perceives patient care, the role of the nurse and the profession influences how that nurse will give patient care on a day-to-day basis. Management factors, including organizational structure, management practices, leadership, and incentives, also influence a nurse's practice. The state of professionalism in nursing care in a given organization, including the type of facilities and equipment, the levels of staffing, and supporting services, are influential in how the nurse functions in a given setting. The manager's role is to evaluate factors that influence productivity of nurses and to work toward achieving an environment in which nurses can apply their knowledge effectively.

Summary

Health-care costs are a matter of concern not only to patients but also to all professionals involved in health-care systems and to the public in general. Controls of costs in the health-care industry can be exerted by governmental forces, by community forces, and by people who work in health-care agencies. Professionals are accountable to their clients, and they are also autonomous in the practice of their selected profession. In this chapter you have been introduced to some of the basic concepts of budgeting and quality assurance. As a manager and a professional you can use this information to develop your expertise in exercising voluntary control over your own practice. This voluntary control is an aspect of professionalism that encompasses not only fiscal control but also control of the quality of services rendered.

Study Questions

1. Interview at least five different nurses, asking each to define quality nursing care. Compare the responses using the following as the basis of comparison:
   a. Terminology used.
   b. Descriptive examples or words used to explain the meaning of terminology used.
   c. Perspective. Did the nurse describe quality nursing care from the perspective of the nurse, the patient, or others?
   d. Similarities and differences in the content of responses.
2. In a group of three to five people, have one person collect data about one patient's hospital bill, including diagnosis, treatment, and costs for hospitalization; if appropriate have another person collect data about the budget of the patient-care unit where the patient was admitted by interviewing the head nurse or by other appropriate means; and have the third person investigate issues of third-party payers in terms of problems encountered in health-care insurance. After compilation of the data, meet to discuss findings and isolate three major issues that you might encounter in budget control when caring for the patient.
3. Conduct a "mini-audit" as a class experiment in which the group writes standards of care to be audited for a selected category of patients. The audit should be limited in scope to one or two aspects of nursing care, and the time frame of the audit should be developed in accordance with situational requisites of the care environment.

4. You have been charged with developing three different plans for setting costs for nursing care given to patients on a medical-surgical patient-care unit. Present your plans to a group, outlining the rationale for each, the costs of each, and the benefits you think would be derived from each plan.
5. Select one procedure or operations method that you have experienced in giving patient care in a health-care agency. Evaluate the procedure or operational task in terms of its efficiency in supporting patient care given by nurses and in terms of cost. As you investigate the procedure, analyze each step to determine whether a different approach would be more efficient or economical.
6. Obtain the staffing schedule for a patient-care unit in a hospital for a period of one month. Evaluate this staffing schedule in terms of:
   a. The mix of nursing personnel
   b. The average number of patients cared for
   c. The types of diagnoses of patients cared for
   d. The acuity of the patients' illnesses
   e. Absenteeism of the nursing staff
   f. Staff turnover (resignations and new employees)

References

1. Argyris, C. Double loop learning in organizations. *Harvard Bus. Rev.* 55:115–125, Sept./Oct. 1977.
2. Bauer, J. C. A nursing care price index. *Am. J. Nurs.* 77:1150–1154, July 1977.
3. Davidson, H. M. The top of the world is flat. *Harvard Bus. Rev.* 55:89–99, March/April 1977.
4. Greene, R. *Assuring Quality in Medical Care.* Cambridge, Mass.: Ballinger, 1976.
5. Lovdal, M. L. Making the audit committee work. *Harvard Bus. Rev.* 55:108–114, March/April 1977.
6. Stevens, B. J. What is the executive's role in budgeting for her department? *Hospitals* 50:83–86, Nov. 16, 1976.

Suggested Reading

Brown, B. (Ed.) Quality assurance and peer review. *Nurs. Adm. Q.* 1:9–50, Spring 1977.
Brucker, M. C., and Reedy, N. J. Quality assurance—an overview. *JOGN Nurs.* 6:9–14, May/June 1977.
Byrd, J. M. Peer review for quality charting. *Superv. Nurse* 8:25–27, July 1977.
Chalef, M. N. (Ed.) *PSRO Journal Articles.* Flushing, N.Y.: Medical Examination Publishing, 1977.
Clark, B. B., and Lamont, G. X. Accurate census forecasting leads to cost containment. *Hospitals* 50:43–48, June 1, 1976.

Cohn, S. S. Audit enhances patient's environment. *Hospitals* 51:61–62, May 1, 1977.

Curtin, L. Human rights and professional responsibilities. *Update On Ethics* 1:1, Aug. 1977.

Davidson, S. V. S. *PSRO Utilization and Audit in Patient Care*. St. Louis: Mosby, 1976.

Davis, A. I. Measuring quality: Development of a blueprint for a quality assurance program. *Superv. Nurse* 8:17–26, Feb. 1977.

Doughty, D. B., and Mash, N. J. *Nursing Audit*. Philadelphia: Davis, 1977.

Froebe, D. J., and Bain, R. J. *Quality Assurance Programs and Controls in Nursing*. St. Louis: Mosby, 1976.

Fuller, M. E. The budget. *J. Nurs. Adm.* 6:36–38, May 1976.

Gosfield, A. *PSROs: The Law and the Health Consumer*. Cambridge: Ballinger, 1975.

Holle, M. L. Retrospective nursing audit—is it enough? *Superv. Nurse* 7:234, July 1976.

Housley, C. E. Budgeting at the supervisor's level. *Hosp. Top.* 54:6, March/April 1976.

Jelinek, R. C., and Dennis, L. C. *A Review and Evaluation of Nursing Productivity*. DHEW PHS, HRA, BHM, Division of Nursing. DHEW Publication number (HRA) 77-15, Nov. 1976.

Lachner, B. J. The cost accountability of the CEO and board. *Hosp. Prog.* 58:60–63, Aug. 1977.

Laros, J. Deriving outcome criteria from a conceptual model. *Nurs. Outlook* 25:333–336, May 1977.

Lohmann, G. A statewide system of record audit. *Nurs. Outlook* 25:330–332, May 1977.

Longest, B. B. *Management Practices for the Health Professional*. Reston, Va: Reston, 1976.

Marram, G. The comparative costs of operating a team and primary nursing unit. *J. Nurs. Adm.* 6:21–24, May 1976.

Marriner, A. Budgets. *Superv. Nurse* 8:53–56, April 1977.

McNally, F. Nursing audit: Evolution without pain. *Superv. Nurse* 8:40, June 1977.

Nelson, C. W. The administrator's role in quality assessment and control. *HCMR* 2:7–17, Winter 1977.

Pearson, B. D. Nursing implications of what price health care? *Nurs. Dig.* 4:51, Winter 1976.

Phaneuf, M. C., and Wandelt, M. A. Quality assurance in nursing. *Nurs. Dig.* 4:32–35, Summer 1976.

Proceedings: Conference on Professional Self Regulation. USDHEW, PHS HRA, DHEW Publication No. (HRA) 77-621, June 1975.

Schaefer, M. J. Forecasting and resource allocation in educational administration. *Nurs. Outlook* 25:256–270, April 1977.

Schulz, R., and Johnson, A. C. *Management of Hospitals*. New York: McGraw-Hill, 1976.

Singer, J. P. Flexible budgeting techniques provide tool for cost control. *Hospitals* 51:45–49, July 1, 1977.

Thompson, J. D. Curriculums must address issues in practice milieu. *Hospitals* 51:73–76, Oct. 1, 1977.

Wallace, R. F., and Donnelly, M. Computing quality assurance costs. *Hosp. Prog.* 56:53–57, May 1975.

Watson, A., and Mayers, M. Evaluating the quality of patient care through retrospective chart review. *J. Nurs. Adm.* 6:17–21, March/April 1976.

Whittaker, A. C., and Holmes, S. L. Man hour budgeting: A refinement of managerial control. *Hosp. Top.* 54:14–16, Jan./Feb. 1976.

II. The Challenge
of Management

The preceding chapters serve to give the reader a cursory view of factors that influence nursing management. This view enables the nurse to form a perspective of the implications of management. Involvement in thoughtful practice of management expands this perspective so that the nurse eventually accumulates a fund of knowledge and experience that gives greater meaning to this cursory view.

When one accepts the commitment to manage patient care, one simultaneously accepts a challenge. This challenge is to participate in developing nursing practice in accord with the social and economic requisites of patient care. Because nursing practice in hospitals is structured, beginning staff nurses are tempted to accept the security of the structure. It is possible to perpetuate the structure in vogue at the time of initial employment through formation of habits and familiarity with secure routines. This perpetuation is not always compatible with sound management practices in a changing environment.

The wide spectrum of patient needs, ranging from acute care to maintenance of health, requires flexibility of nurses. The scope of abilities of nursing staff members also demands flexibility. Therefore, managers must continually question the relevance and practicality of their actions. Management is a continuous process of adaptation.

What seems fixed or stable in nursing today may not be appropriate in the future. The challenge of management is multifaceted and involves answering questions such as:

How should patient care be defined today? In the future?

How should the nursing staff be organized for best advantage?

What tools can be devised to assist nurses?

Your challenge is to become a realistic manager who can deal with the priorities of the present while forging ahead into the future.

The following chapters offer the reader concepts and principles of management that can be employed to ensure that staff members get the job done while experiencing job satisfaction.

The first chapter in Part II deals with motivation. Managers face dual challenges for motivation. They must motivate themselves and nurture the motivation of staff members. As with management, motivation is a continuous process. People need stimulation to improve their abilities, and they vary in the degree of independence they assume. Managers set the tone for staff attitudes by making sure that all staff members have positive experiences in which they are successful in giving patient care. If the staff is successful, the manager is also.

Additional chapters emphasize concepts and principles that can be utilized to ensure staff member job satisfaction and management's goal of quality patient care. Skills in delegating, communicating, interviewing, appraising, teaching, introducing change, and disciplining are presented in a form easily adapted to any nurse-patient setting.

6. Motivation

In order for the nurse to guide and direct staff members, the nurse must first understand the nature of human behavior and understand why people act as they do.

To understand another person, we must know how he feels about himself. His self-image will influence his behavior. A person's self-concept is acquired from childhood experiences and from the feedback he receives from his achievements. A person's behavior is purposeful, and the manager needs to be perceptive in understanding why the staff members are behaving as they are. The successful leader learns the reasons behind the behavior and takes the necessary steps to correct undesirable behavior.

Individuals attempt to fulfill their wants, drives, and needs. The word *motive* implies action to satisfy a need. Further discussion of these concepts follows.

Maslow's Hierarchy of Human Needs

The psychologist A. H. Maslow has developed a theory of human motivation that has been widely accepted [6]. According to Maslow, our needs can be arranged according to priorities into a hierarchy, with physical needs being the "lowest" and most basic, followed in ascending order by security, social, egotistic, and self-actualization needs, as illustrated. In this hierarchy, a higher need does not motivate until the lower, more basic needs are first satisfied, but once a lower-level need is satisfied, it no longer motivates.

Thus, once our need for food, shelter, clothing, and protection from danger is met, we become relatively more concerned with higher needs. Once our desired standard of living is attained, our social needs are motivators, followed by our needs for esteem and respect. The highest need—that which motivates after all other needs have been met—is the ultimate form of accomplishment, self-actualization, which has been described as total fulfillment of the self in making the most of one's potentials. A person moving up the hierarchy may reverse direction and move downward if his lower-level needs are threatened. Once the need is satisfied it no longer serves as a motivator of behavior.

This hierarchy serves as a framework to many contemporary theo-

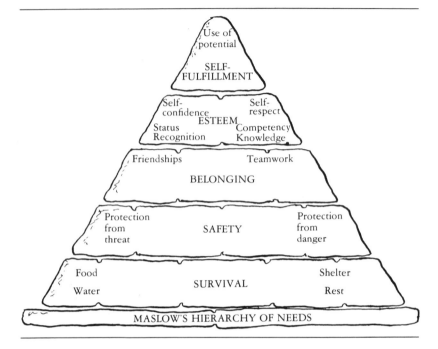

MASLOW'S HIERARCHY OF NEEDS

ries of motivation. It can be further illustrated by the following discussion.

SURVIVAL NEEDS

At the base of the hierarchy are the needs for survival. These are the biological needs of all men for food, water, protection, and rest. These are the lowest-level needs but become the first in importance when threatened.

Most of us have secured these basic needs. Our patients, however, may have these needs thwarted. Hunger can have a dominating influence on a patient's behavior after a day or more of being without food. A patient with chronic renal failure who is on a strict fluid restriction often finds thirst to be such a strong drive that he seeks extra water, even though he knows that it is harmful.

SAFETY NEEDS

Safety needs are fear-based needs for protection against danger, threat, or being deprived of something considered necessary. In the working situation this need may be manifested in workers' demands for tenure, saving and retirement plans, or forms of insurance. A nurse may feel threatened when she does not feel qualified to care for a complex patient. A patient may feel threatened and insecure when placed in an involuntary dependency relationship or when faced with a frightening diagnostic test such as a sternal bone marrow biopsy. A nurse's aide in training may feel psychologically threatened when faced with something new, unfamiliar, or unknown.

Safety needs usually do not become a dominant motivator unless the individual is seriously threatened or endangered, but then they may take over completely. We have read of panic during fires when many people unreasonably attempt to satisfy their individual safety needs at the same time.

BELONGING NEEDS

Once survival and safety needs are satisfied, they cease to motivate behavior. People are social animals and are motivated by the need to belong and to be liked and wanted. They want friendship and often associate with others for companionship. An employee who has an unsatisfactory home life may find that the relationships with fellow employees provide a large part of the social-need satisfaction. Workers who belong to small, integrated work groups often have higher morale than those who work alone. Teamwork helps to build morale. Most people like to help others and to be helped by others when they need it. An individual usually adjusts his behavior to meet the norms of the group.

The Hawthorne studies [8] initiated in 1927, which were conducted on 20,000 workers, pointed out dramatically that the need to be accepted and liked by one's fellow workers was at least as important as and perhaps more important than economic incentives in determining how the individual performs on the job. The workers restricted their production output (to their own detriment from the standpoint of financial gain and promotion) in order to gain acceptance from their fellow workers. The studies also showed how workers resist being put into competition with their fellows and tend, consciously or unconsciously, to band together to resist anything from management that might appear a threat to the individual.

A nurse may be confronted with a group of aides who find greater satisfaction in meeting their group norms—for example, taking extended coffee breaks—than in being more productive in their nursing functions. Greater work output by one of the aides may result in that aide's being rejected by the other aides.

ESTEEM NEEDS

Once the social (belonging) needs are met, esteem needs become the motivators of behavior. These needs include the desire for self-confidence, independence, self-respect, achievement, competence, and knowledge. Esteem needs also include a desire for status, recognition, appreciation, and respect from others. These needs are rarely fully satisfied, and an individual will continue to seek indefinitely for greater satisfaction of these needs. For many people, the need for respect and recognition from others is more important than the need for self-respect.

This fourth level of needs is especially prominent among successful managers, professionals, highly skilled workers, and those with a high need for achievement.

SELF-FULFILLMENT NEEDS

The highest need at the top of the hierarchy is self-fulfillment or self-actualization. These are the needs for fulfilling one's potential, for continual self-development, and for being creative in the broadest sense of the term. Maslow describes the self-actualizing person as one who has the following qualities [5]:

1. Superior perception of reality
2. Increased acceptance of self, of others, and of nature
3. Increased spontaneity
4. Increased problem-solving ability
5. Increased detachment and desire for privacy
6. Increased autonomy, and resistance to enculturation
7. Greater freshness of appreciation, and richness of emotional reaction
8. Higher frequency of peak experiences
9. Increased identification with the human species
10. Changed interpersonal relations
11. More democratic character structure
12. Greatly increased creativeness
13. Certain changes in the value system

All the needs overlap and the lowest needs never disappear. We must always eat, sleep and take refuge from the weather, and no one can think of self-actualization if worried about belonging. These levels are interdependent and overlapping, each higher need level emerging before the lower needs have been satisfied completely. In our society, most people tend to be partially satisfied in each need area and partially unsatisfied. Most individuals tend to have more satisfaction at the lower need levels than at higher need levels.

ADDITIONAL MOTIVATING FACTORS

In addition to basic needs, a person is strongly motivated by the interests, attitudes, and values that he has acquired. Even within the same social milieu there is considerable variation in the abilities, attitudes, and temperaments of people. People react to praise, criticism, promises, and frustration very differently. One assignment may challenge one individual but frustrate another individual. As managers we can be alert to notice and remember the wishes and preferences of our staff. Attitudes, biases, and prejudices should be understood and taken into consideration in nurse-patient contact, as illustrated by the following examples.

1. A nurse's aide was especially interested in caring for patients with colostomies; thus, she was motivated to give good care when assigned to a colostomy patient.
2. A strained, uneasy relationship existed between an Arab doctor and his Jewish patient that prevented the patient from feeling that the physician was genuinely concerned about his welfare.
3. A nurse who was very opposed to alcohol or common law marriage was very judgmental in giving care to a patient who was married by common law to an alcoholic.

Other Theories of Motivation

In addition to the widely accepted theory of Maslow's hierarchy of needs, there are three other important theories of motivation. One has been formulated by psychologist Frederick Herzberg [3]. It is a theory of work motivation rather than a general human motivation theory. Herzberg's researchers asked workers to tell them about events at work that resulted in improved job satisfaction and about events that decreased job satisfaction. When the results were tallied, the factors resulting in increased job satisfaction were labeled as *motivators* because they were effective in motivating the individual to superior performance and effort. These factors were achievement, recognition, work itself, responsibility, and advancement. Another group of factors labeled *hygienic* or *maintenance* factors focused on discontent with the work situation. These included environmental factors (such as working conditions), company policies, administration, supervision, salaries, and interpersonal relations.

The hygiene factors are preventive. If the organization provides them, it will prevent the workers from getting sick of work. But to get the workers to do creative, satisfying, responsible work, the organization must provide them with the motivators.

The healthy worker likes a balance of both hygiene and motivator factors. He wants a pleasant environment, but at the same time he needs to accomplish and create.

If the hospital concentrates on supplying hygiene factors and neglects the motivators (interesting work, responsibility, on-the-job growth, self-improvement opportunities, recognition), then the hospital workers are going to seek the hygiene factors.

Another helpful way of classifying needs for application on the patient-care unit is to categorize needs according to the way they can be satisfied. We can place them into three categories:

1. Needs satisfied away from the hospital
2. Needs satisfied in the hospital environment
3. Needs satisfied through giving patient care

When the hospital administration stresses vacation days and bonus checks, it is attempting to satisfy employees' needs away from the hospital. The hospital that provides coffee on the unit for the nurses is attempting to satisfy needs in the working environment. This helps to make the environment pleasant, but it does not provide direct motivation in rendering patient care. It is the third category, that of satisfying needs through the giving of patient care, that should be emphasized if managers wish to provide positive motivation to staff to work harder. Basically, the physical and security needs are satisfied off the job, social needs are satisfied through personal contacts around the job, and egotistic needs are chiefly satisfied through the job.

David C. McClelland [7], a Harvard psychologist, has investigated the achievement motive in people. The subjects for his experiment were shown pictures and were to tell a story about each picture. This technique revealed what the subjects thought about when they were not required to think about anything in particular. If one spends time thinking about doing things better, psychologists say he has an achievement orientation (*n Achievement*). If one spends time thinking about family and friends, he has an affiliation orientation (*n Affilia-tion*). People with a strong need for power (*n Power*) want to command attention, get recognition, and control others. Most people possess some of each, but there are people who lean more in one direction.

McClelland's research has shown that achievement-oriented people tend to translate their thinking into action. They place great demands upon themselves, are persistent, realistic, and believe in moderate risk-taking. Evidence suggests that high achievers have come from parents who set moderately high achievement goals but who were warm, encouraging, and nonauthoritarian in helping them reach these goals. McClelland points out that individuals who score high in achievement motivation are motivated by the love of accomplishment, interest in their work, and by success itself.

No matter how high a person's need to achieve may be, he cannot succeed if he has no opportunities, if the organization keeps him from taking initiative or does not reward him if he does.

The third theory is behavior modification. B. F. Skinner [9] is a leading proponent of the behaviorist school of psychology, which holds that behavior is caused primarily by externally induced stimuli. He thinks that man and his environment are the focus for behavior and that all behavior is shaped and maintained by its consequences. A person does something because of the reinforcement he received the last time he behaved in a similar way. If the outcome of his action pleases him, he is likely to repeat the action. A reinforcer is something that increases the probability of a behavior's occurring again.

There are three types of reinforcement:

1. Punishment reinforcement
2. Extinction or neutral reinforcement
3. Positive reinforcement

Punishment is used to decrease the behavior. Skinner argues against punishment. Extinction consists of applying a neutral stimulus after the behavior occurs. Positive reinforcement is the most recommended by Skinner since it increases the likelihood of a desired response. Informing staff members of how they are doing is a form of reinforcement. Positive reinforcement may consist of a smile or a nod of approval. It should come as soon after the behavior as possible.

Morale and Productivity

Recent research shows that there is no simple correlation between morale and productivity. There can be high morale with low productivity or low morale with high productivity. Morale can be defined as the total satisfaction a person derives from his job, his work group, his boss, the organization, and his environment. It is affected by the person's personality and pertains to the feeling of well-being, satisfaction, and happiness.

Rensis Likert [4] claims that the relationship between morale and productivity for complex and varied work tends to be moderately high. When the job performance depends upon the individual or team, then those workers who like their job are more likely to be motivated to produce. Much recent behavioral research has demonstrated that when the leader and the team are highly work motivated, then team members' satisfactions and attitudes are often positive.

The ideal system of work motivation is to provide opportunities for need-satisfaction through doing the job itself. This necessitates developing staff commitment to the objectives of the health-care agency. Ideally people will exercise self-direction and self-control in working for objectives to which they are committed. This emphasizes openness and trust, supportive supervision, and participation in decision-making.

IMPORTANCE OF TASK

How can the nurse provide satisfaction to the staff in the category of providing patient care? Let us look at some of the dimensions of the egotistic needs. One of man's strongest needs is the need for a sense of accomplishment—that the work is important. Therefore, the importance and value of the task to be done must be emphasized. If the aide who is to give a patient an enema is told that the enema is an important preparation for an x-ray that is of diagnostic value for the patient, the aide will be better able to see the importance of the task. Prevention of skin breakdown should be stressed in helping an aide see the importance of keeping the incontinent patient clean. There are many unpleasant tasks in nursing that nurses must do; understanding their value helps promote a feeling of satisfaction when the task is accomplished.

SENSE OF ACHIEVEMENT

Staff members also need to feel a sense of achievement in their tasks. They need some way of measuring their progress. Everyone wants to know, How am I doing? People like feedback even when there is no reward or penalty attached to failure or success. We generally receive feedback from our patients. For example, a patient might say, "That backrub feels so good," or "I feel much more comfortable now that I have had my medication." Other patients, however, are unable to tell the staff how they feel. It may be an aphasic patient or a very withdrawn patient that the staff is caring for. In these cases it is important for the professional nurse to apprise the staff on how they are meeting the patient's needs.

SENSE OF CREATIVITY

Another egotistic need is that of enjoying the sense of creativity that springs from doing something well, from being "on top" of the job. People like to imagine that their jobs require unusual skill and as a consequence tend to exaggerate the job's importance. If you have ever observed one hospital maid showing a new hospital maid her job, you will probably have seen her stressing its complexity. The professional nurse should acknowledge the skills of those doing jobs of less status than her own. The maid may be pleased to have cleaned four rooms to be ready for the new admissions of the day; the orderly may tell you that he has helped ambulate ten patients; and the maintenance person may be pleased to announce that the side rail on bed A in room 303 is now fixed. All of these employees like to feel that their job is important, that they have done it well, and that they had special skills that made it possible to complete the task. Managers must not fail to use the creative abilities of the staff, for they like to use their initiative and imagination.

Motivation and Productivity

Generally, people in our society have a genuine desire to work and to be productive in their employment. Then why do we see employees who loaf and at times go out of their way to avoid working? Usually such behavior indicates that the individuals are dissatisfied with their job, with their supervisor, or with the work place, or feel that they have been treated unfairly. It is important to identify the underlying problem that is keeping a staff member from being a productive member of the team and attempt to correct it.

SATISFYING HIGHER-LEVEL NEEDS

As previously stated, a satisfied need is no longer a prime motivator of behavior. This must not be overlooked in nursing. For example, consider the aide who was interested in caring for colostomy patients.

Her interest might have stemmed from the intense desire to learn as much as possible about colostomy care. If she is assigned time and time again to the colostomy patients, however, she may have her need met, and it will no longer serve as a motivator. She must now be provided with opportunities to meet higher-level needs. If her higher-level needs are ignored, she will feel deprived. This can be manifested by frequently taken sick days or decreased effectiveness on the unit.

Managers cannot provide staff members with self-respect or esteem, but they can create conditions that foster rather than hamper the satisfaction of these needs. Managers need to know in which situations an individual staff member seeks recognition. To tell an aide that she gave an enema well when she has given fifty enemas well may mean little to her. Managers need to recognize the areas that are a challenge to the aide and then must praise the performance of the task that was difficult to accomplish.

As mentioned earlier, the professional nurse sometimes encounters an unproductive staff member. Staff members are motivated not so much by what you want them to do as by their own desire to get along as best they can in the situation they perceive. It may be that you are overmanaging staff members by too narrowly defining anticipated behavior and making too many decisions for them. By making minimal and confining demands on staff members' abilities and by placing all decision-making in the leader's hands, managers provide little opportunity for responsibility, self-reliance, or independence. Staff members need a sense of pride and accomplishment from their work, not a childlike role that is neither stimulating nor dignifying.

GELLERMAN'S THEORIES OF POSITIVE MOTIVATION
Dr. Gellerman [2], a noted manager, has written management theories describing three methods which have been found to have a positive motivational effect. They need to be applied selectively, as they may not be effective in all cases.

One method is called *stretching;* this is the assignment of tasks that are more demanding (in difficulty level, not necessarily in terms of time or effort) than you believe your staff capable of handling. This enhances the likelihood that staff members will use more of their potential to experience the satisfaction of achievement and will develop a desire for more of it. This method should be used sparingly and infrequently. It must not be used as a continuous motivational method.

A second method is *management by objectives;* that is, giving the staff members rather broad direction as to how they perform a task, provided they accomplish the end goal.

The third method is *participation;* that is, seeking the staff's comments and suggestions prior to making significant decisions affecting their work. Research seems to indicate that the power of participation to motivate persons stems primarily from its capacity to give a feeling of personal worth through the recognition that the individual receives from others in the group.

OTHER MOTIVATIONAL CONSIDERATIONS

Dr. Mortimer R. Feinberg [1], an industrial psychologist and personnel consultant, states that the best way to motivate subordinates is to show them that you are conscious of their needs, ambitions, and fears and recognize them as individuals. In other words, identify what level of needs staff members are attempting to satisfy before conversing with them, and then plan your interaction with them to be in tune with their level of needs. This will show them that you recognize and understand what is important to them.

There are actions to be avoided if you are concerned about motivating the staff. Do not belittle a staff member. You may have had a teacher in school who belittled students if they gave a wrong answer, and before long the students stopped volunteering answers. Do not criticize a staff member in front of others. Do not get so preoccupied with your thoughts that you fail to listen to your staff members with undivided attention. Do not play favorites or make exceptions because of personal preference for a staff member. Other staff members will resent it and lose motivation. Do not vacillate in making a decision. Being wishy-washy shows your lack of confidence, and staff members will then lack confidence in you.

There are positive actions the manager can cultivate in order to motivate staff. Communicate to the staff your standards so that they have a goal and a guide. Be consistent in these standards. Recognize your own biases and prejudgments in order to prevent them from altering your objectivity. Keep staff members informed of their performance and inform them of changes that may affect them. Go out of your way to help the staff to develop, and take responsibility for the staff members. If one of them fails, you, too, fail in part. You have probably heard the remark "Oh, that happened on the evening shift" as a response to a reprimand by a physician that a patient's need was not met. In contrast, the head nurse who assumes responsibility for patient care around the clock must have nurse leaders who assume responsibility for actions of their group members. Encourage staff members to be independent by encouraging them to solve problems, show initiative, think creatively, and ask pertinent questions. Be willing to learn from others; acknowledge ideas, suggestions, and proposed changes that are brought to you. Demonstrate confidence; if you have doubts about your head nurse, your nursing supervisor, or the director of nurses, review them alone. Do not review them with subordinates. Exhibiting doubts to staff members disheartens them and tends to lessen their confidence in you. Allow freedom of expression. Staff members should be allowed to make their jobs interesting by doing it their own way as long as the principles are followed and the desired results attained. Be tactful and courteous.

There are many factors that motivate individuals. To be an effective leader, one needs to understand individual staff members' needs and to help them attain satisfaction in their work. Provide them with more interesting work, more responsibility, and the opportunity for achievement. Managers need to tap the staff's valuable resources in planning and carrying out patterns of patient care.

Study Questions

1. Choose a staff member with whom you are well acquainted to illustrate what types of things the leader needs to understand about the staff member in order to promote motivation.
   a. Can you give an example of how well you understand one of the staff members by describing the member's interests, wants, and needs?
   b. What happens when those needs go unsatisfied?
   c. How can you create conditions that will encourage this staff member to attain satisfactions on the job?
   d. What specifically can you do to make this staff member's job more satisfying?
2. Staff members have the following needs. Discuss how you can manage staff members to see that these needs are met. Give specific examples of what you can do.
   a. Belonging needs.
   b. Sharing in planning the group goals.
   c. Attaining meaningful goals.
   d. Knowing clearly what is expected so as to work confidently.
   e. Challenging duties and responsibilities that are within range of abilities and that contribute toward reaching the goals.
   f. Seeing that progress is being made toward the goals that *we* have set.
   g. Keeping informed. What the staff is not *up* on, it may be *down* on.
   h. Confidence in the leader, based upon fair treatment, of recognition when it is due, and trust.

3. As a group exercise, relate to one another the specific things that motivate you as an individual. What do you respond to?

References

1. Feinberg, M. R. *Effective Psychology for Managers.* Englewood Cliffs, N.J.: Prentice-Hall, 1965. Pp. 122–142.
2. Gellerman, S. W. *Motivation and Productivity.* New York: American Management Assn., 1963. Pp. 105–121.
3. Herzberg, F. *Work and the Nature of Man.* Cleveland: World Publishing, 1973. Pp. 91–111.
4. Likert, R. *The Human Organization.* New York: McGraw-Hill, 1967. Pp. 53–77.
5. Maslow, A. H. *Toward a Psychology of Being* (2nd ed.). Princeton, N.J.: Van Nostrand, 1968.
6. Maslow, A. H. (Ed.) *Motivation and Personality* (2nd ed.). New York: Harper & Row, 1970. Pp. 35–58.
7. McClelland, D. *The Achieving Society.* Princeton, N.J.: Van Nostrand, 1961. Pp. 36–62.
8. Roethlisberger, F. J., and Dickson, W. J. *Management and the Worker.* Cambridge: Harvard University Press, 1939. Pp. 511–524.
9. Skinner, B. F. Where Skinner's theories work. *Business Week,* December 2, 1972, pp. 64–65.

Suggested Reading

Axne, S., Boniger, G., and Dodson, D. Staff motivation through a self-help design. *Superv. Nurse* 7:65, Oct. 1976.
Chopra, A. Motivation in task-oriented groups. *Nurs. Dig.* 5:80, Fall 1977.
Ford, R. N. *Motivation Through the Work Itself.* New York: American Management Association, 1969.
Gellerman, S. *Motivation and Productivity.* New York: American Management Association, 1963.
Gellerman, S. *Management Motivation.* New York: American Management Association, 1968.
Herzberg, F. One more time: How do you motivate employees? *Harvard Bus. Rev.* 46:53, Jan./Feb. 1968.
Holloway, R. C. Management can reverse declining employee work attitudes. *Hospitals* 50:71, Oct. 16, 1976.
Livingston, J. S. Pygmalion in management. *Harvard Bus. Rev.* 47:81, July/Aug. 1969.
Mager, R. and Pipe, P. You really oughta wanna or how not to motivate people. *Nursing '76* 6:65, Aug. 1976.

Marriner, A.   Motivation of personnel. *Superv. Nurse* 7:60, Oct. 1976.

McClelland, D. C., and Winter, D. J.   *Motivating Economic Achievement.* New York: Free Press, 1969.

Nusinoff, J. R.   How to motivate your employees toward more effective patient care. *Hosp. Top.* 54:50, Mar./Apr. 1976.

Roche, W. J., and MacKinnon, N. L.   Motivating people with meaningful work. *Harvard Bus. Rev.* 48:97, May/June 1970.

Skinner, B. F.   *Beyond Freedom and Dignity.* New York: Knopf, 1971.

7. Development of Staff

In the majority of hospital nursing situations, the nurse cannot meet all the patient needs alone. Limited time and energy prevent the nurse from being all things to all patients. Professional nurses most frequently provide patient care with the assistance of subprofessional nursing personnel and paramedical personnel. Thus, the nurse becomes involved in delegating aspects of patient care to others. Before the care can be delegated, the nurse must know that the tasks can be performed well by the staff. Often, this involves informal teaching and training to perform tasks.

The objective of this chapter is to discuss management principles used in helping people to develop their potential in the working environment. The reader will be presented with behavioral and environmental aspects affecting learning, principles of learning, teaching techniques, problems that may prevent development of staff, and forms of adult education.

The influence the professional nurse has on a staff member depends upon their relationship as individuals. Emotional attitudes of the teacher and student are extremely important. The nurse needs to be trained to recognize and deal with normal emotional factors that prevent learning from occurring. The nurse needs to be aware of staff needs in order to identify and communicate with staff members and must show confidence in the staff's capacity to perform. They, in turn, must respect the nurse as a person with ability and integrity, worthy of authority. They must believe that their leader has the knowledge and skills of a professional nurse and represents model conduct. This does not mean they need to be friends, or even that they need to like each other. We like people for social reasons; we can respect people, however, for their honesty, their courage, and their ability.

The Helping Relationship

Carl Rogers defines a helping relationship as one "in which at least one of the parties has the intent of promoting the growth, development, maturity, improved coping with life of the other" [8]. This definition of a helping relationship can apply to the nurse-manager's relationships with staff members.

From research done on students at the Massachusetts Institute of Technology [3], we find some very helpful principles in understanding the dynamics of helping relationships. These principles can be broken down into five key areas:

1. The *task* or problem around which the helping relationship develops
2. The helper's *motivation* (achievement motivation—n Achievement; power motivation—n Power; affiliation motivation—n Affiliation) and his *self-image*
3. The *receiver* of help and the receiver's motives and self-image
4. The *environment* and *psychological climate* in which the helping activities occur
5. The information *feedback* which occurs during the helping process

THE TASK

The task can be placed on a scale. At one end of the scale the receiver of help takes a passive, uninvolved role. At the other end of the scale is education. The helper avoids using his special skills and knowledge to solve the task and instead works with the learner's frame of reference to increase the learner's ability to solve the problem. This method can help the learner the most but may cause frustration if the learner wants an immediate solution to the task.

THE HELPER AND RECEIVER OF HELP

The personal characteristics of the helper and learner are very important in the helping relationship.

The power motivation of the helper and the learner determines how much they will attempt to influence and control each other. The helper needs to deal with a tendency to feel "superior." The learner needs to overcome feeling weaker or dependent. These feelings must be dealt with in order for a helping relationship to develop.

The affiliation motivation of the helper and the learner determines how much they will be concerned about intimacy and understanding. The helper needs to know how the learner understands and perceives the problem. A lack of affiliation puts them in two different worlds. Too much affiliation can produce pressure toward conformity and sympathy, which may result in the helper's losing perspective on the problem and the learner's losing respect for the helper's expertise.

The achievement motivation of the helper and the learner determines how concerned they will be about accomplishing the task or solving the problem. The two need to agree on a mutually acceptable goal.

There is an interaction among motives in any helping relationship. If the power motivation is too high, the helper and learner can get preoccupied with controlling one another at the expense of understanding each other or accomplishing the task. High achievement motivation can cause the helper and learner to orient themselves to accomplishing the task without giving attention to the interpersonal aspects of influence and understanding needed for the learner to solve the problem on his or her own. "Here, let me help you" may result in the helper's pushing the learner aside, thus leaving the learner nearly as ignorant as before in regard to solving the problem. High affiliation motivation can result in the accomplishment of the task's taking a back seat to intimacy and understanding between the learner and helper.

Thus, for helping relationships to occur, moderate levels of achievement, affiliation, and power motivation in the helper and learner are necessary. The dynamics of the helping relationship are such that influence, intimacy and understanding, and a concern for task accomplishment are all necessary for effective help to take place; yet excessive concern in any one area can lead to deterioration of an effective helping relationship.

The self-image and attitudes of the helper and the learner are also important to the helping relationship. The learner must see himself as capable of improvement and must be willing to receive help. The helper must see himself as capable of helping without being a "know-it-all." The helper must be willing to influence and at the same time have empathy for the feelings of the person he is helping.

THE ENVIRONMENT AND PSYCHOLOGICAL CLIMATE
Behavior is a function of both the person and the environment. Comfort of surroundings, freedom from distraction, and the individual's perception of the environment all influence the learning process.

FEEDBACK
The last factor in the helping relationship is information feedback. Two aspects of information feedback are important. First, there is the source that controls information. Feedback can be controlled by the task, as in the case of programmed instruction, or by the receiver of

help, as in self-research methods, or by the helper, as in traditional teaching methods.

The other important aspect is the nature of the feedback. Most learning theorists have concluded that in the long-run reward is more effective than punishment. Carl Rogers, in his concept of unconditional positive reward, places heavy emphasis on the importance of positive feedback to the learner. "I find that the more acceptance and liking I feel toward this individual, the more I will be creating a relationship which he can use. By acceptance I mean a warm regard for him as a person of unconditional self-worth—of value no matter what his condition, or his feelings. . . . This acceptance of each fluctuating aspect of this other person makes it for him a relationship of warmth and safety, and the safety of being liked and prized as a person seems a highly important element in a helping relationship" [8].

EFFECTIVE HELPERS, INEFFECTIVE HELPERS, AND NONEFFECTIVE HELPERS

An effective helper is one who, in an environment where giving help is appropriate, attempts to help others, while the others see this help as significant and important to them. The ineffective helper attempts to give others help, but these others do not regard the help as important. The nonhelper does not attempt to help. The MIT experiment showed that ineffective helpers scored much lower on n Affiliation than did effective helpers or nonhelpers. Ineffective helpers scored much higher on n Power than did effective helpers or nonhelpers.

As far as self-image is concerned, the nonhelpers are different from both the effective and ineffective helpers in that they describe themselves as more passive, democratic, not cynical, submissive, followers, guarded, quiet, timid, not influential, inarticulate, self-conscious, and preferring to listen. The general picture is one of an accepting, democratic person who lacks the self-confidence to influence others.

Ineffective helpers describe themselves as organized, impatient, open, and superior. These adjectives summarize a person extremely self-confident with impatience and lack of interest in others.

The effective helpers consistently place themselves between the ineffective and nonhelpers. They are self-confident without being overbearing, and they score moderately in achievement, affiliation, and power.

These results focus on the two types of help that are doomed to failure—the brash, overconfident, superior approach, which places the learner on the defensive, and the timid, hesitant, passive approach, which may raise questions about the helper's qualifications and lead to a lack of confidence in the helper. The results of the research also showed that the effective helpers gave more positive feedback and ineffective helpers gave more negative feedback.

To summarize the experiment, the helping relationship is best viewed as one involving a complex interaction of at least three motives—n Achievement, n Affiliation, and n Power. Effective helpers appear to be those individuals who score moderately on these three motives. Similar moderation appears in the self-image of effective helpers. They are not as brash and overconfident as ineffective helpers nor as timid and self-conscious as nonhelpers. The feedback that is received from effective helpers tends to be more positive and less related to control issues than feedback from ineffective helpers.

Understanding Viewpoints of Others

Effective communications are of paramount importance in the nurse's relationships with staff. However, a common problem frequently exists in our communications with others. We have a natural tendency to evaluate, to judge, to approve, or to disapprove the expressed opinions of the other person. The primary reaction is to listen to another's expressed opinion and evaluate it from one's own point of view [7]. An example could occur during a patient-care conference when a nurse states that a patient seems to be exaggerating his discomfort. Almost invariably your reply will be approval or disapproval of the attitude expressed. This tendency to evaluate another's opinion can be a major barrier to interpersonal communications.

Rogers [7] states that we can solve this problem by avoiding the evaluation and instead seeing the attitude or idea from the other person's viewpoint. This is not as easy as it may seem. A way to test your ability to understand rather than to evaluate is to try the following experiment. The next time you have an argument or heated discussion with a friend or with a group, institute this rule: You may speak your opinion only after you have restated the last speaker's opinion to his satisfaction. This means you must achieve his frame of reference.

Too many managers fail to listen intently when communicating with staff. Do you tap your fingers on the desk, allow yourself to answer the phone, or fidget when a staff member is talking with you? You need to hear the staff's feelings as well as their words. Feeling has its source in emotions, and emotions are the most potent catalyst of action. Feelings, if not allowed to escape, can develop into forces of anxiety and frustration that erode morale and efficiency and produce incompetency.

Asking Staff for Opinions

How do we know if our perceived attitudes foster suggestions from the staff? Are you listening only for what you want to hear? Are you making patient-care decisions without the opinions, counsel, and assistance of the staff? If you do more than half of the talking at a patient-care conference that includes a group of staff members, it is a good bet that you fall into this category. Are you really interested in getting the advice or suggestions of staff members? The risk involved in not getting counsel from the staff is that you are failing to provide them an opportunity to develop. Another important risk is damage to morale. Patient care is the end product at stake. A good rule to follow is to seek staff's counsel on major patient-care decisions. If a decision has already been made, solicit advice on how to implement it.

The relationship the leader has with staff members depends upon the leader's attitudes and feelings toward them. If the nurse accepts and respects them as individuals and has a positive and helpful attitude, a nonthreatening environment is promoted in which staff can learn and develop. This can be termed a "climate of confidence." The staff members must feel that they are approved of as individuals, that their strengths and weaknesses are recognized, and that they are important persons doing an important job.

Candor with Staff

If you promote an open atmosphere, your staff will not feel inhibited about talking freely with you. Frankness, honesty of opinion, and forthrightness are the key words. This means being honest with them when you do not know the answer to their questions. Tell them you do not know rather than brushing off the question or giving a feeble reply. It means tolerating their questions about your decisions. They should sense that you do not become defensive when questioned. It means openly accepting criticism of your behavior. It may be better to hear things that hurt from time to time than not to get the true feelings of the staff. This is difficult behavior to develop for the leader who lacks self-confidence and for the autocratic leader. Perhaps such an attitude is difficult for the most competent leader at times. It is a goal, however, toward which all should work.

Here, again, make a self-check. Next time you are in a conference discussing a controversial subject, make a note of how often ideas contrary to your own are advanced. If they come up rarely, or not at all, you probably have failed to create an open environment.

Influence of Manager's Expectations

What a manager expects of staff members and the way they are treated largely determine their performance. Staff members, more often than not, do what they believe they are expected to do [5]. This is similar to other patterns of human behavior. We have seen the relief of pain from placebos. The patient's response was related to what was expected. In a series of scientific experiments, Robert Rosenthal of Harvard University has demonstrated that a "teacher's expectation for her pupil's intellectual competence can . . . serve as an educational self-fulfilling prophecy" [9]. An experiment conducted with 60 preschoolers of equal ability compared the performance of pupils of teachers who had been led to believe their students were slow learners to that of pupils of teachers who had been led to believe their students had rapid learning ability. Pupils of the second group learned much faster.

Staff members can usually sense the leader's attitude toward them; they know whether or not the leader believes they can meet expectations. Too frequently, however, managers are unaware of the feelings they transmit to others. The nurse's standards of patient care are revealed by the example the leader sets. If the nurse gives thorough skin care to patients, for example, staff members will be inclined to give the same quality of care. Nurse-leaders therefore transmit their expectations by their behavior as well as by what they say.

An important aspect of the ability to transmit high expectations is the leader's self-confidence in the ability to motivate and develop the staff. If the leader has doubts about the ability to stimulate the staff members, the leader will expect less of them. An executive has been quoted as saying, "Your administrative success will be in direct proportion to your subordinate's belief of your belief in him" [6].

Managerial expectations have the greatest effect on new employees who have not yet formulated their attitudes on how well they can perform in a nursing situation. This is very significant when one thinks of the generally high turnover rate of nursing personnel. One can see the importance of having new personnel placed under the leadership of a nurse with high standards and high expectations of staff. The staff members' self-confidence will grow, their capabilities will develop, and they will be more productive as a result of good leadership.

Principles of Learning

Teaching is another necessary part of developing staff members to their fullest work potential. Every contact you have with staff can be an opportunity to teach. Some attention to the principles of learning is helpful. Most of these have been formulated by psychologists [2, 4, 10].

Learning can be defined as that human process by which skills, knowledge, habits, and attitudes are acquired and utilized in such a way that behavior may be modified. Psychologists, primarily through experimentation, have developed a number of important principles of learning. These are equally pertinent for application by training directors who administer programs, classroom instructors who teach employees, and supervisors who train employees on the job.

MOTIVATION

The individual must be motivated to learn. He needs to be aware of the inadequacies of his present behavior, skill, or knowledge and have a clear idea of the behavior he needs to attain.

Adequate motivation is essential to the success of any learning experience. People are goal-oriented in their behavior. They will exert themselves to fulfill a felt need. Learning is effective when the trainees perceive that they can satisfy some goal through participation in a training program. The staff members must see the need to improve their abilities and job performance in order to benefit from attempts to develop their potential.

Both rewards and punishment play a powerful role in motivation to learn. A reward for a desired response serves to stimulate a repetition of that behavior. Mild punishment is effective if it is immediate and if the learner understands the reason for it. This must be handled very judiciously, for punishment may cause the learners to resent or fear the instructor so much that they cannot concentrate upon learning the work.

Generally, people will learn to behave in a desired way if they understand the reasons for the desired behavior and if they are rewarded for such behavior.

Leaders can help motivate the staff by giving new and challenging assignments, by delegating authority, and by rotating tasks. Assignments should be planned so that they are meaningful to each individual.

REINFORCEMENT

Related to motivation is the need for reinforcement. For learning to take place, the individual must receive some encouragement or reward. In many cases the reward need not be tangible. The learner needs to experience some feeling of progress, either through the leader's comments or through self-observation that the job was well done. Praise for progress is more effective than punishment for mistakes made. Most people have only limited tolerance for failure. Learners must be made aware of their failures, but the ability to tolerate failure should be a function of the success achieved and the degree to which correct behavior has been reinforced.

FEEDBACK

In order for reinforcement to be effective in improving performance, there must be feedback, or knowledge of results. Research experiments have demonstrated that people learn faster when they are informed of their accomplishments. Such knowledge should be automatic, immediate, and meaningfully related to the task at hand. The learners need to know how their performance measures up to the desired standard. When learners have made a mistake, they need to recognize why and how they went wrong and how close they came to doing it correctly. All too frequently positive feedback is not given. The feedback you give should be given in a nonthreatening environment if possible. In other words, do not correct your staff in the presence of the patient or others unless it is absolutely necessary for patients' well-being. Praise, too, should usually be given in private. When criticizing, criticize the action, not the individual. Feedback should be provided as soon as possible after the performance is observed.

LEARNING BY DOING

Learning is most efficient when the learner is actively involved rather than passively listening to a description. The most economical and practical training method should be selected for the type of desired learning. Much patient-care related training has taken place on the job under the direction of the employee's or student's immediate supervisor. Simulated learning experiences and modern technology are now being used to develop the learner's active involvement in developing competency. Motor activity directly stimulates the higher mental processes, such as learning [1]. The greater the number of senses involved, the more effective the learning. Doing rather than just seeing or hearing also means that the individuals are more likely to devote more of themselves to the task; they become more involved in the learning process. The difference between knowing a principle and making it work must be learned by performing. Permit mistakes to be made when they will cause no harm. Mistakes are then corrected, and the correct behavior reinforced.

SPACED REPETITION

Many experiments have shown that learning periods distributed through time are more efficient than single, sustained attempts. Repetition serves to inhibit forgetting. Without practice, learned skills gradually disappear.

LEARNING BY PARTS

Learning is enhanced when the total process or skill to be learned is divided into small segments, each of which can be mastered in a sequence until the total task is learned. Whether or not this is possible depends on what is to be learned. For example, the nurse's aide in training may have three weeks to master the skills of giving a patient morning care. The skills involved may include taking the patient's temperature, pulse, and respirations, giving the patient a bath, making a bed, and helping the patient with ambulation and with the use of a bedpan. If each of these tasks can be taught separately rather than attempting to teach them all at once, learning can be enhanced.

LEARNING BY MASTERING LARGE SEGMENTS

Learning is inhibited if the segments to be mastered are too small. Integrating fragments into a whole activity as a smooth, continuous process becomes extremely difficult. Whenever possible, the learner should try to master as a single unit all those activities that must be performed in a smooth, continuous sequence, as a complex pattern cannot be learned until all its parts are practiced simultaneously. Separate practice of the parts can improve the learner's skill in each one, but it cannot teach the learner the total pattern. An example of this principle would be teaching a practical nurse how to insert a Foley catheter. The procedure encompasses principles of asepsis, cleansing techniques, anatomy, positioning, and assembling equipment. All these aspects of the total procedure need to be practiced in a smooth, continuous sequence.

PROVIDING THEORY

Learning is faster and can be better applied to new situations if the learner understands the principles involved. In nursing situations the employee who knows the "whys" behind the skill is better able to transfer knowledge to new situations. If the staff is to develop insight into new problems that arise during the course of rendering patient care, a more basic understanding of activities than that provided by "this-is-how-you-do-it" training needs to be achieved. Logical training is more effective than rote training in nursing. Therefore, staff members should be taught sufficient theory to understand the principles and reasons underlying their work and to cope successfully with the general types of problems they may encounter.

GEARING LEARNING TO THE INDIVIDUAL

All human beings can learn. The effective teacher sees that each learner has different needs and abilities and so must be taught in a different way. The learner must secure satisfaction from the learning. In other words the training must seem useful to the learner. Teachers have a strong inclination to make people over into their own image. This temptation should be avoided and should be replaced by understanding that each learner must achieve results within the framework of the learner's personality and motivations.

When teaching, the nurse-manager must start at the student's present level. Do not assume that the learner knows or does not know something. To determine what the learner knows, ask a question that requires an explanation rather than one that must be answered by "yes" or "no." You waste your time and the staff's time explaining something they already know. Observation of the staff members working with patients and with fellow workers will give you insight and valuable information as to their level of performance.

We must not judge performance solely on results, with little or no consideration of how the results were obtained. The results do not always justify the means. You can observe the action directly or utilize questions to determine how the results were obtained.

LEARNING MOTOR SKILLS

If the skill to be taught is a motor skill, the instructor begins by showing and explaining the supplies and equipment needed. The activity is then performed by the instructor. If it involves steps, the procedure should be broken down into logical components and explained. Next the learners should practice the procedure. They should understand what they are doing and be able to explain the activity. The instructor should provide guidance and feedback. The learners must know if their performance is progressing properly or not. A rest period should follow the practice period. Distributed practice periods are more fruitful than prolonged and concentrated practice.

LEARNING CONCEPTS AND ATTITUDES

This process is much more complex than learning motor skills. There are many ways to learn ideas and attitudes. We can learn by trial and error, by personal experience, by reading and observing, or by listening and talking with others.

Preservation of Staff Initiative

It can be a temptation, when observing a staff member involved in patient care, to pitch in and take the initiative. For example, a staff member may be giving care to a comatose patient. If you want to help, refrain from initiating such care as turning the patient or giving range of motion exercises. When being aggressive in initiating care, you tend to stifle the initiative of the staff. Your help is very supportive, but refrain from "stealing the thunder" from your learner. The staff will derive much more satisfaction in initiating the plan of care and then receiving your help in carrying it out.

Exploring Problems Through Questions

The ability to ask good questions is essential in teaching. Good questions help the learner gain insight and understanding. You do not want your questions to seem threatening or authoritarian; rather, your intent is to explore the problem and in so doing bring greater understanding to the learner. The same holds true for questions brought to you. There is a temptation to derive personal satisfaction from being an authority and to exhibit your knowledge by answering the question. This may be necessary in situations where an immediate answer is needed. If time permits, however, the question can be used as a learning process. By asking the learner questions leading up to a solution, the leader can help the learner determine the answer. For example, the staff may ask you, "Mr. Smith wants some milk. May he have it?" You can reply with questions such as: What kind of diet is he on? Is that included in a low-fat diet? Is he having any tests done today?

If a staff member comes to you with a solution to a problem that you believe will not work, do not answer with a "That will not work because . . ." This is not teaching by the use of problem-solving. Instead, attempt to get the staff member to explain how the solution was determined. You can ask questions such as: What are some advantages and disadvantages? or What alternatives did you consider, and why did you reject them? It is by answering these questions that problem solving is accomplished.

Demonstration

Skill in demonstration is another effective tool in teaching. Prior to the demonstration you should prepare staff members by discussing what is to be demonstrated. Here again, utilize questions to keep learners actively involved, to determine how much of the activity is already understood, and to find gaps in knowledge that will need special emphasis. The demonstration should be as lifelike as possible. For example, "Resusci-Anne," a training manikin, is a very lifelike tool for teaching heart-lung resuscitation. At the conclusion of your demonstration, have the learners demonstrate back to you, if this is feasible, and have them explain what is happening and why. Learning is reinforced when the learner repeats the procedure soon after it is learned, and retention is increased by repetition. It is useful to plan to have the learner perform the skill at the earliest possible opportunity, and have the learner explain to you how the procedure will be done just prior to doing it. The demonstration or return demonstration should be followed by an analysis and evaluation to ensure the learner's complete understanding. Guard against expecting the learners to repeat the demonstration exactly as you originally performed it. A grasp of the principles is more important. Let the staff members develop the methods most suited to their abilities and limitations.

Potential Impediments to Teaching Role

Some nurses hesitate to utilize these principles of staff development. They claim it is faster to do a job themselves than to show someone else how to do it. They believe there just is not enough time. Others fail in this management role because consciously (or unconsciously) they lack self-confidence or adequate nursing knowledge. Some nurse-teachers fail to disclose all their "tricks of the trade," fearing competition. Others cannot communicate with staff because of an age barrier or a personality clash—for example, when a new graduate nurse leads a group of employees who have been at the hospital five or ten years.

For several reasons the staff may not accept help from the professional nurse. The staff may feel knowledgeable and thus become very sensitive to suggestions and criticism. The staff may lack self-confidence in their ability to do the job, or the staff may fear the professional nurse. Poor communication often proves to be the reason for failure. Resistance to change also hampers development.

It is important to identify the preceding problems. Factors preventing development of individuals or groups rendering patient care have their effect on the quality of patient care given. Interest, ingenuity, and fresh approaches must be developed by the group to solve problems of patient care.

In-Service Education Programs

Hospitals with in-service education programs often provide a variety of adult education programs. Some hospitals provide employees with the teachers and time needed to complete courses for a high school diploma. Other hospitals offer special courses such as speed-reading. Employees of some hospitals are given an opportunity to take college courses with the hospital paying part or all of the tuition.

In-service education, a form of adult education, is a means of keeping staff members informed of the many advances and changes in medicine, nursing, and management. M. Shanks [11] writes that an in-service program has four components:

1. Orientation
2. Skill training
3. Continuing education
4. Leadership training

ORIENTATION

Although proper orientation is easily and often neglected, it is essential for ensuring that new employees get off to the right start. Orientation is the guided adjustment of the employee to the organization and the work environment.

Orientation programs are advantageous to both the hospital and the employees. The hospital administration seeks to create favorable attitudes about its goals, policies, and personnel. A well-run orientation program may minimize the likelihood of policy violation, discharges, resignations, grievances, and misunderstandings.

In most instances the employee is partially oriented to the hospital before starting work. Such orientation began with the employment interview and from the reputation the hospital has earned. After the employee is hired, the orientation progresses with both the personnel department and the nursing personnel playing key roles.

The personnel department needs to orient the newcomer by explaining the pay, pay increases, promotion opportunities, holidays, vacations, and benefit plans. It should also train the nursing personnel in the performance of their orientation responsibilities.

The role of the orienter (this may be the head nurse) is to make the newcomer feel welcome. This person should review the job description with the new employee, introduce the other staff members working on the unit, and conduct a tour of the patient-care unit and its facilities.

The following is a list of important content information and actions that may be included in an orientation program.

1. Hospital history, policies, practices
2. Hospital services
3. Hospital facilities
4. Organizational structure
5. Employee responsibilities to the hospital
6. Hospital responsibilities to the employee
7. Pay
8. Rules of conduct
9. Tour of the hospital
10. Work schedules
11. Collective bargaining agreement and union relationships
12. Benefit plans—life insurance, medical, hospitalization, pension, unemployment
13. Safety program

14. Training or educational opportunities
15. Promotion policy
16. Introduction to fellow employees
17. Establishment of a feeling of belonging and acceptance, showing genuine interest in new employee
18. Employee appraisal system
19. Work assignment

SKILL TRAINING

These programs serve to train the nonprofessional hospital employee. The nurse's aide, for example, needs to be taught the skills required in the hospital's job description. Referring to the sample job description on page 207, one sees that the nurse's aide must know how to do a variety of functions, including taking vital signs, giving enemas, hematesting stools, and collecting specimens. These skills should be learned and practiced under the supervision of the instructor either in a classroom or on the patient-care unit. To leave initial teaching and supervision of aides to staff members is unfair to both the aides and the staff members unless provision is made for a special "mentor system." The staff members' primary concern is the patient, whereas an instructor in the classroom can give full concern to the aides-in-training.

CONTINUING EDUCATION

Continuing education is either mandatory as a requisite for relicensure or voluntary in almost every state. In most states there are stipulations about the types of programs that qualify for continuing education. Some of the continuing education programs must be obtained from sources other than the institution that employs the nurse, but many employing agencies conduct programs that can be used to meet a portion of the total continuing education requirements.

Continuing education is also supported by the Joint Commission on Accreditation of Hospitals. The Nursing Services section of the Accreditation Manual published by the JCAH includes a requirement that there must be continuing training and educational programs for nurses in the hospital. Both the American Nurses' Association and the National League for Nursing have published information about continuing education. The American Nurses' Association publication *Continuing Education in Nursing: Guidelines for Staff Development* contains information about goals for staff development programs, the organization of staff development departments, the roles of personnel, and evaluation of programs. Staff development terminology is also defined.

Some staff development programs include a continuing education component designed to provide learning experiences for nurses that include content and skills different from those learned in basic educational programs in nursing but that are general to the practice of nursing. Staff development programs also include learning experiences specific to the practice of nursing in a given health-care agency. The types of programs specific to an agency include orientation programs and in-service education. Orientation consists of an introduction to the role and expectations of nurses in a given agency. In-service education is designed to increase the knowledge and skills of nurses employed by an agency in relation to their roles and job descriptions in that agency. Continuing education in the hospital can be done in a wide variety of ways. For example, it may encompass a televised education program such as "Surgical Repair of an Aortic Aneurysm"; it may be an on-the-unit drill of the procedure for cardiac arrest; it may be a formal presentation by a guest or by a member of the medical or nursing staff; or it may be an informal lecture by a technician on the use of a new piece of equipment. The key to a successful continuing education program is to survey the employees to learn their wants and needs for the program. For example, to teach professional nurses how to make a bed might be folly; there would be no interest or need. A questionnaire may be used to gain suggestions from staff members for in-service educational programs. Once a program is scheduled, the nurse-leaders should encourage as many staff members as possible to attend. This may involve scheduling the program to be presented at different hours in order to reach nurses of the three shifts and to maintain nurses on the unit with patients during the program.

LEADERSHIP OR MANAGEMENT TRAINING
This aspect of in-service education is generally concerned with the preparation of professional nurses for leadership or supervisory positions. The authors believe that such training can be beneficial to all registered nurses.

Each patient-care unit not only can participate in the agency's in-service educational program but can also have an educational program on the unit. Staff members on an orthopedic unit may be interested in specific aspects of orthopedics that a delivery room nurse might find less useful. Once a subject of interest is found among staff members, the subject can be studied in a variety of ways. One or more staff members can research the subject at the library and bring the information back to the others; a specialist in the subject can be asked to lead an informal question-and-answer discussion; or a film may be shown on the patient-care unit. It is also helpful if staff members can attend conferences and courses and share their information with those who did not attend. For example, the Hawaii Heart Association presents an annual three-day conference on cardiovascular nursing. Those nurses able to attend gain a great deal educationally.

With such a variety of means for continuing education, all staff members should be able to gain new knowledge. Not only should all levels of the nursing staff be considered, but also personnel on the evening and night shifts.

As M. Shanks states so well, "In-service education cannot force individuals to learn, but it can emphasize the need to learn and can be the stimulus for personal and professional development . . . It is rapidly becoming a successful method towards improving care for patients" [11].

Group Session

The following questions are written for group discussion. Get a group of classmates or friends together to discuss these questions if you do not have an opportunity to answer them in a classroom session.

1. Have two people role play a teaching situation. Have one assume the role of the professional nurse and the other the role of a nurse's aide. The nurse is to teach the aide how to get a paraplegic patient from the bed to the wheelchair. Have the other members of the group observe the interaction between the nurse and the aide and evaluate the teaching situation in terms of:
   a. Relationship between the nurse and aide
   b. Utilization of learning principles
      (1) Motivation
      (2) Reinforcement
      (3) Feedback
      (4) Learning by doing
      (5) Spaced repetition
      (6) Learning by parts
      (7) Learning by mastering large segments
      (8) Providing theory
      (9) Gearing learning to the individual

(10) Learning motor skills
(11) Learning concepts and attitudes
c. Utilization of techniques in questioning
d. Utilization of techniques in demonstrating

Additional situations that could be used are positioning a comatose patient, putting a patient through range of motion exercises, and feeding a C.V.A. patient.

2. Have members of the group reflect and share with the others two memorable events in their working experience: (1) What moment stands out in your memory as being the most satisfying experience? (2) What moment has been the most dissatisfying experience? Analyze why the experience was satisfying and why the contrasting experience was dissatisfying. What implications can you derive from this to apply to your role in developing staff?
3. Are any members of the group having difficulty with staff members who are not functioning at their potential? If so, describe the individual's behavior and attitudes to the group. Utilize this example to investigate the problem and to derive possible solutions. Have the group approve a strategy to be used in future interactions with the staff member. Have the nurse-leader utilize these suggestions and report back to the group on how effective the solutions were in the actual situation. This situation and others of similar types can be followed in as many group discussions as necessary until the problem is solved.
4. Select an emotional and controversial issue that members of the group can use to argue conflicting positions. Divide into opposing groups and begin to debate. At a given time, stop to analyze how much communication took place. Return to the debate, and this time utilize the suggestion of Carl Rogers as noted in this chapter, "You may speak your opinion only after you have restated the last speaker's opinion to his satisfaction." Were you able to see a difference in how much real communication took place?
5. Identify attitudes and habits that you have seen on your patient-care unit that are barriers to communication. What communication habits do you have that you would like to change?
6. Did your orientation program to the health-care agency or school communicate high standards? Was there one person in particular who stood out in your mind as a role model?

References

1. Allport, G. The psychology of participation. *Psychol. Rev.* 52:117, May 1945.
2. Hilgard, E. (Ed.) *Theories of Learning.* National Society for the Study of Education 63d Yearbook. Chicago: University of Chicago Press, 1964. Pp. 1–360.

3. Kolb, D. A., and Boyatzis, R. E. On the dynamics of the helping relationship. In *Organizational Psychology: A Book of Readings* (2nd ed.). Englewood Cliffs, N.J.: Prentice-Hall, 1974.

4. Leavitt, H. *Managerial Psychology*. Chicago: University of Chicago Press, 1964. Pp. 65–80.

5. Livingston, J. S. Pygmalion in management. *Harvard Bus. Rev.* 47:81, July/Aug. 1969.

6. Myles, M. *The Growth and Development of Executives*. Boston: Division of Research, Graduate School of Business Administration, Harvard University, 1950.

7. Otto, C. P., and Glaser, R. O. *The Management of Training*. Reading, Mass.: Addison-Wesley, 1970.

8. Rogers, C. *Carl Rogers on Personal Power*. New York: Delacorte, 1977. Pp. 3–27.

9. Rosenthal, R., and Jacobson, L. *Pygmalion in the Classroom*. New York: Holt, Rinehart & Winston, 1968. Pp. 174–182.

10. Skinner, B. F. *Science and Human Behavior*. New York: Macmillan, 1953.

11. Shanks, M., and Kennedy, D. *The Theory and Practice of Nursing Service Administration* (2nd ed.). New York: Blakiston Div., McGraw-Hill, 1970. Pp. 248–264.

Suggested Reading

Chokrieh, A. In-service education, leadership and management. *Nigerian Nurse* 8:37, July/Sept. 1976.

Munn, Y. L. How to get it and use it in nursing today. *Nurs. Adm. Q.* 1:95, Fall 1976.

Nelson, M. A. Building a better team. *Nursing '77* 7:65, July 1977.

Schaefer, M. J. The knowledge worker. *J. Nurs. Adm.* 7:7, April 1977.

8. Introducing Change

Today's nurses are seeing many changes in the field of patient care and health-care agency management. New medications, new equipment, and new methods of treatment are being introduced to the health-care scene at a rapid rate. We like to think that we keep up to date in a field where last year's knowledge may be obsolete today. Some changes we may welcome readily—for example, lighter, easier to handle cardiographic equipment or computerized medication selection. But we tend to resist the changes introduced by management that affect our interpersonal and job relations. Why do we resist these? Because they tend to threaten the security of the patterns to which we have grown accustomed.

In order for health-care agencies to meet the increasing demands for patient-care services, changes in management of personnel must occur. The ability to introduce such changes with a minimum of resistance is a key managerial skill. This chapter deals with people's reactions to change on the job and how change can be introduced in an acceptable way.

Why Individuals Resist Change

Automation may make an employee feel that he will no longer be needed and may therefore lose his job. In hospitals we have seen automation in the transportation of food trays from the kitchen to the patient, in the use of the computer for staffing, and in the use of television to enable the nurse to visualize the patient in his room.

A worker may resist the change of assignment of duties. For example, a licensed practical nurse may be so accustomed to helping ambulate patients in the rehabilitation department that she resents a new job of planning recreational activities for patients that will require different duties. It does not take long for an individual to develop a routine in an everyday work situation. Learning new ways which have been brought on by change requires energy that individuals may resent putting forth. In other words, it is easier not to change.

Another factor in the worker's resistance to change is the uncertainty that change brings. The reason for the change may not be understood. The uncertainty may be helped by explaining the purpose for the change and answering the worker's questions.

Changing work procedures and systems and introducing new equipment may also upset the interpersonal relationships established prior to the new system. For example, two aides on the evening shift always divided the unit in half according to room numbers for their giving of patient care. When the student nurse-leader attempted to arrange assignments according to patient-care needs, she met with much hostility and resentment from the two aides. They had developed their own work pattern and resisted change that would affect their interpersonal work relationships.

Fear of failure may also cause resistance to change. Individuals may feel that they are doing their jobs well now and that the change will alter their ability to work as well.

Employees may view change as having to take orders. If the so-called orders come from supervisors who have little contact with the staff members or from a student nurse-leader who is not one of the regulars, the staff members may view and resent the change as coming from an outsider.

Unions are also likely to resist change unless management consults with them either formally or informally. More and more health-care employees are being organized into unions.

The Nature of Resistance

The key to the problem is to understand the true nature of resistance. What employees resist is usually not technical change but social change—the change in their human relationships that generally accompanies technical change. Resistance is usually created because the people introducing the change are so preoccupied with the technical aspects of the new idea that they do not see how the change will affect social relationships.

We need to think of change as having both a technical and a social aspect. The technical aspect of the change is the making of a measurable modification in the physical routines on the job. The social aspect refers to the way those affected by the change think it will alter their relationships to the organization. The nature and size of the technical aspect of the change does not determine the presence or absence of resistance nearly as much as the social aspect.

Therefore, nurse-managers need an in-depth, detailed understanding of the specific social arrangements that will be sustained or threatened by the change or by the way that it is introduced.

Many changes take place without resistance. People who work

closely together often swap ideas to make their work easier. Because they work so closely and because they initiated the ideas, these changes are not threatening.

By contrast, if the change is initiated by the agency administration or by someone higher up in the hierarchy who is not a part of the working unit, the changes are more likely to be resisted. We may sometimes wish that the validity of the technical aspect of the change were the sole determinant of its acceptability. The fact remains, however, that the social aspect is what determines the presence or absence of resistance.

Even after the plans for change have been carefully made, it takes time to implement them fully. Time is necessary even when there is no resistance to the change itself. If the staff members feel that they are being pushed and are not allowed enough time to implement the change, they will begin to resist it.

An attitude that may cause trouble is assuming that the change will result in resistance. Staff members will sense this attitude, and you will probably get the resistance you are anticipating as a result.

When resistance does appear, do not think of it as something that needs to be overcome. Instead, think of it as a signal that something is going wrong. Paul Lawrence [1] uses an interesting analogy. He says that signs of resistance in a social organization are useful in the same way that pain is useful to the body as a signal that some bodily functions are getting out of adjustment.

The resistance, like the pain, tells you something is wrong. You need to find out what is causing the pain. To take a pain killer or to try to stop the resistance without first finding out the cause of the pain or resistance will not take care of the basic problem. Therefore, when resistance does occur, you need to listen carefully to find out what the problem is.

It may be a technical reason that is causing the difficulty. More likely, however, the problem will be a result of threatened established social arrangements for doing work.

If efforts to create positive attitudes towards the change fail before the change is implemented, then the nurse-manager may decide to enforce the change regardless of the attitudes. The nurse-manager then relies on cognitive dissonance to dissipate the resistance. The concept of cognitive dissonance asserts that when a person is required to demonstrate a given behavior consistently, his or her attitudinal patterns are apt to become favorable to the enforced behavior [2]. In other words, as the person behaves in the required way, he resolves the conflicts between his attitudes and his behaviors. By doing the required activity, the individual will soon rationalize that activity's desirability.

How We Get Staff Members to Accept Change

No change can be successfully carried out unless logical and psychological foundations have been established. Generally, the logical foundation is built well but the psychological aspect is less well designed. If the psychological foundation—the one concerned with staff members and their possible reactions to the proposed change—is not well designed, staff member resistance may follow.

A positive approach to building the psychological foundation for change has been outlined by Nathaniel Stewart [3]. He calls for the following measures:

Identification
Reassurance
Communication
Participation
Mutual interest
Follow-through

IDENTIFICATION
This refers to having the staff members themselves identify with the problem. Employees must first see and feel the need to change. For example, the Waterton Hospital administration decided that each patient-care unit should change from a verbal report to oncoming shifts to the use of a taped report. Prior to the change, 4 North, a hectic, disorganized floor, took an average of one hour to complete reports between shifts. The staff members considered this unsatisfactory and were eager to try the tape recorder to see if this would lead to better utilization of nursing time. Three North, however, was able to give a 20-minute report verbally that was prompt and complete. The staff members on 3 North, therefore, had difficulty identifying with the change introduced by the use of the tape recorder.

REASSURANCE
Industrial psychologists agree that employees will seek to protect the job satisfactions that exist and will be apprehensive of any proposal that may infringe on established satisfactions. This anxiety must be alleviated prior to acceptance of the change. The following situation

illustrates this point. The intensive care unit and coronary care unit functioned as separate units with separate staff members but were adjoining geographically at Waterton Hospital. A plan was devised for merging the staffs of the two units to achieve greater flexibility in staffing patterns. Prior to the change there were days during which the coronary care unit had three nurses caring for only one patient while the adjacent intensive care unit had three nurses caring for ten patients. The new plan would allow nurses to float between the two units when needed. The staff nurses in the intensive care unit were very anxious as they felt unqualified to interpret electrocardiogram monitor strips. The coronary care unit nurses were also anxious about the proposed change. These anxieties needed to be recognized and alleviated by those introducing the change. Fortunately, the nursing management of Waterton Hospital saw the need for in-service education to precede the change so that the nurses would have class preparation for new experiences in patient care. This was a necessary aspect of reassurance.

COMMUNICATION

If change is desired, it must be explained carefully and thoroughly. Important changes affecting staff members should be communicated face-to-face in a personalized way, not via an intercom or a printed handout. It is a must that the communications precede the change. Staff members need to be thoroughly informed and have their questions answered in advance of a proposed or pending change. Background and reasons for the change should be communicated to staff members. As health-care agencies grow bigger and more complex, the need to communicate in understandable language must not be overlooked.

Organizations have grapevines that spread news and rumors rapidly. To prevent unwarranted speculation from growing, management should keep staff members informed throughout the planning, introduction, installation, and follow-through of the change.

PARTICIPATION

Participation of staff in the management of change is a psychological and functional asset in management. It is helpful to solicit from staff members their suggestions, views, and criticisms of the proposed change. The communication pattern should be such that staff members talk to each other as well as to the person introducing the proposed change. It is important to encourage the staff members to express themselves. T. A. Wickes [5] points out that getting opinions out in the open so that they can be examined and evaluated is an important, trust-building task. Ideas that get no hearing often seem better to their author than ideas that actually get used. During staff members' discussions, the leader should refrain from asking staff members to "stick to the subject." What may seem to be irrelevant tangents often contain personal and emotional elements that need to be brought out and discussed. Failure to do so may result in staff members dragging their feet instead of cooperating with the change.

Participation will not work if it is used as device to get others to do what you want them to do. Real participation is based on respect. Respect is acquired when the nurse-manager faces the reality that the contributions of the staff members are needed.

Ideas should not be solicited from the staff members if in fact there is no flexibility in the plans for change. Involving staff members deeply in a project and then incorporating nothing of what they had to offer in the plan of action may result in anger and frustration among those staff members consulted.

MUTUAL INTEREST

Proposed change should appear to solve problems at the patient-care unit level as well as in the overall management of the agency. It is helpful to identify how the new changes will benefit staff members as well as management in contrast to the existing system.

FOLLOW-THROUGH

Change often takes time. Time must be allowed for organizational, technical, and human change. Follow-through is needed in each of these areas to detect and correct any weaknesses or difficulties in the change. When playing tennis it is not enough to hit the ball. The stroke must continue past the moment of hitting the ball to the stage called follow-through in order for the ball to sail on target. So too with proposed change. Without follow-through the change may be sent out but may fall off course rather than landing on target. It is necessary to make certain that the solution is really suitable to the problem that prompted the change.

Techniques for Introducing Change

One of the most common and most difficult problems in introducing change is that of bringing in a new nurse to head an already established unit. If the former head nurse was well liked, the new one will have to contend with the staff members' attitudes that the new nurse cannot be as good as the former head nurse. Staff members wonder what changes the new head nurse will make. They may resent the newcomer as an outsider and prepare themselves to reject everything the new head nurse does.

Let us examine this problem and how it was handled in a specific situation. Keep in mind that although the case discusses a new head nurse the same could apply to a new group leader or a new staff nurse who is a group member. The example will illustrate techniques that may be helpful in introducing change in a wide variety of situations.

Mrs. Bennett, head nurse in the intensive care unit, had developed warm relationships with her staff members. The nursing supervisor was afraid that Mrs. Bennett's departure from the head nurse position would have a bad effect on the morale of the staff members. Consequently, the supervisor prepared the way for Mrs. Bennett's departure with great care. The supervisor discussed the problem of a replacement with the registered nurses in the intensive care unit.

When the new head nurse, Miss Fischer, was selected, she was introduced to the staff members at a general meeting. The nursing supervisor announced that Mrs. Bennett would be leaving and went on to say how much she had meant to the unit. Mrs. Bennett spoke of her sadness in leaving and then introduced Miss Fischer, extolled her virtues, and asked the staff members to show Miss Fischer the same cooperation they had given her. Finally, Miss Fischer promised to do her best to follow in Mrs. Bennett's footsteps.

For the next few days Miss Fischer followed Mrs. Bennett around, getting to know the staff members and trying to learn Mrs. Bennett's routine and methods of dealing with people.

Although Miss Fischer decided that she would eventually make certain changes in the intensive care unit, she spent her first few weeks trying to follow the human-relations patterns established by her predecessor. Only after she was fully accepted by the group did she begin making changes.

What techniques were used here to win acceptance for the new head nurse? How might these techniques be used in other situations? Strauss and Sayles [4] outline the following points:

Consultation. The nursing supervisor involved the registered nurses in the selection process and thus substantially increased their acceptance of the final decision.

Introduction. The former head nurse was careful to introduce the new head nurse to all key personnel and to explain the customs of the unit. This helped to prevent the new head nurse from making social faux pas, to integrate her into the social pattern of the organization, and to minimize the amount of disruption caused by the change in command.

Ceremony. The meeting at which the head nurse was introduced and a farewell party for the departing head nurse both served a ceremonial or symbolic function. They formalized the fact of change and helped the old head nurse pass on some of her prestige to the new. The use of ceremony is a public proclamation that, in spite of apparent change, the basic values remain the same.

Avoiding change until acceptance is assured. The new head nurse avoided making changes until she had developed informal social relationships with her subordinates. It is usually wise for new managers to wait before taking action until they know more about the organization and the people with whom they are dealing.

Building on the past. The new head nurse made it clear that she had no intention of throwing out past practices wholesale. As missionaries have discovered, it helps to learn the customs of the people with whom one works. Changes can be introduced more easily if an adjustment is made to the past.

Conclusions

In conclusion, you, the nurse-leader will be involved in changes that you or others in the health-care agency have introduced. Too often we concern ourselves solely with the technical aspect of change and fail to consider the human-relations problem that many changes generate. A seemingly small change may have profound ramifications. Staff members may have vested interests in the old ways; they may fear the uncertainties of the new. People seldom resist change just to be stubborn; they resist because it hurts them economically, psychologically, or socially.

Nurses helping to introduce change need to seek out the reasons for resistance to the change. They need to find out how the change will affect the people involved, and particularly how it affects their interrelationships.

The first step in dealing with resistance is to bring the problems out in the open with two-way communication. Objections and suggestions for modification should be carefully listened to. Some suggestions may not be realistic, but their airing brings them into the open for consideration. Some objections and modifications may be useful, and their acceptance will improve the overall quality of the proposed change.

Group Session

1. How would you personally react to the following situation?

    You have spent considerable time Monday preparing your plan of care for patient A for Tuesday. This preparation included reading his entire chart, studying textbooks about his medical condition, and talking with patient A. On Tuesday morning, you find your assignment has been changed so that someone else is caring for patient A.

    a. What would be your initial reaction?

    b. What factors would help you to accept this change?

    c. What factors would hinder your accepting this change?

2. Analyze times in your life when you had to undergo change. Which changes went smoothly? Why? Which changes did not go smoothly? Why?

3. Which staff members on your unit adjust to change easily? Which ones adjust less easily? Is there a correlation between their adjustment and their needs? What levels of needs (Maslow's hierarchy of needs) are affected by change?

4. Give examples of recent changes introduced on your unit. What were the technical implications? What were the social implications? What were the various reactions by individual staff members? Could the change have been introduced in a way that would have promoted easier acceptance?

5. Plan a hypothetical change for your nursing unit. Outline the steps included in the change. If practical, implement the change on the unit and analyze the results. If this is not practical, role-play with a group the effects of the change. What follow-up measures would you use?

References

1. Lawrence, P. R.   How to deal with resistance to change. *Harvard Bus. Rev.* 32:49–57, May/June 1954.
2. Stevens, B. J.   Management of continuity and change in nursing. *J. Nurs. Adm.* 7:26–31, April 1977.
3. Stewart, N.   Nothing is as permanent as change. *Nation's Business* 47:33, 57–59, Aug. 1959.
4. Strauss, G., and Sayles, L. R.   *Personnel: The Human Problems of Management* (3rd ed.). Englewood Cliffs, N.J.: Prentice-Hall, 1972. Pp. 241–263.
5. Wickes, T. A.   Techniques for managing change. *Automation* 14:84–87, May 1967.

Suggested Reading

Aeschilman, D. D.   A strategy for change . . . the nurse practitioner must develop a workable solution, gain acceptance for the solution, acquire negotiation skills, and develop the reputation as a successful innovator. *Nurse Pract.* 1:121, Jan./Feb. 1976.

Asprec, E. S.   The process of change. *Superv. Nurse* 6:15, Oct. 1975.

Bennis, W. G., Benne, K. D., and Chin, R.   *The Planning of Change.* New York: Holt, Rinehart & Winston, 1969.

Bunning, R. L.   Changing employees' attitudes. *Superv. Nurse* 7:54, May 1976.

Guerin, Q. W.   A functional approach to attitude change. *Manage. Rev.* 59:33, 1970.

Labovitz, G. H.   How to improve your management effectiveness in coping with change. *Hosp. Top.* 52:24, July/Aug. 1974.

Leary, P. A.   The change agent. *J. Rehabil.* 18:30, 1972.

Miller, B.   The manager—roadblock to change? *Manage. Rev.* 50:4–12, April 1961.

Mullane, M. K.   Nursing care and the political arena. *Nurs. Outlook* 23:698, 1975.

Nehls, D., Hansen, V., Robertson, P., and Manthey, M.   Planned change; A quest for nursing autonomy (Minneapolis, Minn. Univ. Hosp.). *J. Nurs. Adm.* 4:23, Jan./Feb. 1974.

Reinkemeyer, A. M.   Nursing's need commitment to an ideology of change. *Nurs. Forum* 9:340, 1970.

Smith, D. W.   Change: How shall we respond to it? *Nurs. Forum* 9:391, 1970.

Soltis, R. J.   A systematic approach to managing change. *Manage. Rev.* 59:2, 1970.

Stevens, B. J.   Effecting change. *J. Nurs. Adm.* 5:23, 1975.

Stevens, B. J.   Management of continuity and change in nursing. *J. Nurs. Adm.* 7(4):26, 1977.

9. Devising and Using a Plan of Care

The professional nurse uses a plan each and every day that patient care is assigned to the staff. This chapter discusses the nurse's role in the hospital in assessing patient needs, planning for these needs to be met by the members of the staff, and supervising and evaluating the patient care rendered. As the nurse formulates the plan for the day, the following questions should be considered, which will serve as a guide in the development of this chapter.

1. What are the general and specific needs of each patient?
2. What are the abilities, interests, and limitations of the staff working today?
3. What is the plan for the day?
4. How can the plan be communicated to the staff?
5. What method of follow-up should be used?
6. How can the effectiveness of the plan be evaluated?
7. What alterations may be necessary in the plan?

The General and Specific Needs of Each Patient

The need for the nurse to know well each of the patients on the unit cannot be overemphasized. The nurse can gain information by reading the patient's chart, by discussing the patient with the patient's physician, the nursing staff, and the appropriate paramedical staff, by talking with the patient's family and friends, and, most importantly, by talking with the patient.

ASSESSING PATIENT NEEDS THROUGH ROUNDS
One of the best ways of getting to know the patients is through nursing rounds. The term *rounds* in this context means seeing the patients for the purpose of assessment. More specifically, the goals of rounds may be to: (1) get to know the patient, (2) give the patient a chance to know the nurse, (3) inform and teach the patient, (4) serve as a liaison between the patient and hospital services, (5) evaluate patient care, and (6) improve communications between the staff and the patient.

Nursing rounds can be accomplished in a variety of ways for a variety of purposes. M. Melody and G. Clark [8] have written of a method of making rounds as an entire team. Their method of rounds takes place after the change of shift report. Rounds at this time are for the purpose of discussing plans with patients, refining preplanned assignments on the basis of changes in the patients' condition or patient preference. On other units the offgoing shift may make rounds with the oncoming shift during the report. The purpose and technique of rounds may also vary with the time of day. A nurse may want to make quick rounds immediately after report to check briefly the current status of all the patients and to make more careful observations of the patients with multiple or critical needs. The nurse may want to make midmorning rounds for the purpose of talking with each patient, to inform patients of tests, or to check how their morning care is progressing. As physicians visit their patients, the nurse may want to go along to communicate to the physician the status of the patient and to learn the physician's findings and plans for the patient. This gives the nurse the opportunity to hear what the physician says to the patient so that the nurse can clarify plans to the patient if necessary, and also helps to keep the goals of the nurse and the physician in agreement. The nurse may make rounds just prior to reporting to the next shift to see if needs have changed and if tests and care have been completed.

There is much information to be gathered during rounds. The position and expression of the patient can indicate how he is feeling. What the patient does or does not say may be an indication of what he is thinking. Equipment must be checked for correct functioning. The current status of dressings and wounds should be checked. The environment should be observed. Does the patient have water? Is the light shining in his eyes? You may need to utilize this time to consult with the patient on the patient-care plan for the day or to answer patient questions. As you enter each room, you should have specific objectives in mind as to what to observe, learn, or discuss while with the patient.

INTERVIEWING THE PATIENT
The nurse should be familiar with interviewing techniques when talking with patients. It is best to develop a system that is comfortable to you rather than using a cookbook recipe of "how to interview" that may result in artificiality. Your primary objective is to get the

patient to talk to you. This requires that you be a good listener. A good listener conveys understanding and interest in what the person is saying. A friendly facial expression and an attentive but relaxed attitude are important. You can also use phrases such as, "Uh-huh," "I understand," or "Could you tell me more?" You may need to steer the conversation tactfully to gain purposeful information about the patient. If you need to ask a question, avoid questions that can be answered with a simple yes or no. Avoid giving an indication that what the patient says pleases or displeases you. Also avoid giving advice; it is better to help the patient work through his own problems. The basic purpose of this nondirect approach is to enable the nurse to determine how the patients see the problem or situation and then to help them think and feel their way through to a solution. This text does not attempt to discuss interviewing in depth. The reader can study interviewing in greater depth by referring to authors [4, 10, 11] who utilize different approaches in the interviewing technique.

OBTAINING INFORMATION FROM OTHERS

Information about the patient can be obtained from the patient's family and friends. Such questions as, "Has he been confused before?," "What types of food does he like?", or "Do you have stairs in your house?" can be helpful in gathering information about a specific patient. Relatives are often relieved to sit with a staff member and talk about their concerns for the patient. By being supportive of the family, one indirectly helps the patient. Research in pediatrics has shown that if a mother's anxiety can be relieved, she in turn is less anxious with the child (who can sense the mother's feelings). The child relaxes as the mother relaxes. Therefore, family and friends can be of help to the nurse not only in giving information about the patient but also in being supportive to the patient.

Patient needs can be brought to the awareness of the staff through conferences. A patient-centered conference draws on the staff members' observations of the patient. Patient problems are identified, and solutions are discussed by the staff. The conference serves as an opportunity for members to share their information about a patient with the rest of the staff. T. Kron [5] discusses the team conference in depth.

In conclusion, one obtains information about patients in many different ways. Leaders must be aware of the various avenues for information and utilize them effectively. To misjudge a patient's need negates the entire plan. Problem-solving must start with a correct definition of the problem. One must therefore *correctly* identify patient needs before proceeding with a plan.

The Abilities, Interests, and Limitations of the Present Staff

The nurse must know what each of the staff members is qualified to do. This should be spelled out in the hospital policy in the form of a job description for each level of nursing personnel. A sample job description is outlined at the end of this chapter. The Nurse Practice Act, which varies from state to state, and the American Nurses' Association's statement of standards are sources of general information. The most reliable information about the staff's qualifications is obtained from observing the patient care the individual staff members give.

This emphasizes the need for the nurse to have frequent personal contact with the staff in order to learn their interests, abilities, and limitations. The nurse may learn that Miss Cousins, RN, has developed a good rapport with the patient Mrs. Long and would like to continue caring for her. Mr. Monk, LPN, may work best with male patients. Miss Kahn, a nurse's aide, may not like caring for the unconscious patient. The nurse who does not yet know the staff well can get helpful information about them from the head nurse. If there are students or working-in-training personnel on the unit, their learning needs should be known. Discussions with the instructor and reading the students' course objectives are means of ascertaining what these students are allowed to do and what experiences would be most helpful for them.

Once this information is obtained, the nurse can continue on to the next step in planning patient care.

The Plan for the Day

We now know the needs of our patients and the abilities of the individual staff members who are to meet the patient needs. We now must arrange a plan for the interaction of patients and personnel to take place. Ask yourself the following questions:

1. What do you want to achieve today? What results need to be obtained?

2. What is the order of the priorities for the day? What can wait, and what must be done today?
3. Who is going to do it?
4. How should they do it?

UTILIZING TIME

Let us look at you, the leader, as a starting point. How can you best utilize your time? A good place to start is by writing a list of things to do in their order of importance and then crossing them out as they are accomplished. People always postpone the difficult, and that is why it is important to accomplish the high-priority items first. Why is this helpful? Because many people fall into the bad habit of wasting time by giving too much of their time to the things they like to do or find easy to do. The list helps you to stick with your goal.

A head nurse who makes unoccupied beds in her free time seems to be wasting talent that could be better spent with patients or staff. The nurse who grabs the phone when it rings rather than waiting for the secretary to answer is also losing valuable time. It helps to think of what your time is worth in dollars. If you are getting paid $8.50 per hour and the secretary is getting $3.00 per hour, then do a job worth the $8.50—not the $3.00 an hour job. Time is too precious to waste. If you have to wait at the end of the phone or for a staff member to appear, do not use the time idly. You can jot down observations of the day, make revisions in the plan, or be thinking of aspects of patient care.

One aspect of utilizing your time well is to know when a job has been completed. The vast majority of people let go of each task far short of the completion point. We need to look at the beginning and the end of each task. For example, we have encountered patients who put their call lights on at frequent intervals. If the nurse answers their verbal requests only and considers the job completed, the light may go on again. The patients may have additional needs to identify and meet. They may be fearful, angry, insecure, or uncomfortable. By the staff's not meeting patient needs the first time the light is answered, valuable personnel time and patient satisfaction are sacrificed. Partial completion of a task may result in having to go back to the patients over and over again.

BUDGETING TIME

Time should be budgeted. If a conference is scheduled to last 20 minutes, then conclude it at the end of twenty minutes. Do not allow sidetracks to prolong it beyond the budgeted time. One management author [2] suggests a time budget that is arranged in four broad areas: routine work, regular work, special assignments, and creative work. The nurse may find that routine work includes checking that patient menus have been collected, that doctors' orders have been checked off, and that laboratory tests have been completed. Try delegating as much of this work as possible to a staff member. You should concentrate on doing your regular work—passing medications, going on patient rounds, meeting complex patient-care needs—in about two-thirds of your time. This would leave time for accepting special assignments and for doing creative work on the unit. For example, you may want to set up a new method for giving tracheostomy care, plan a conference with the physical therapy department on how a patient is progressing, or have a conference with a patient and the public health nurse.

The more systematic you are, the more effective you will be in the use of your time. You need to make a conscientious effort to avoid

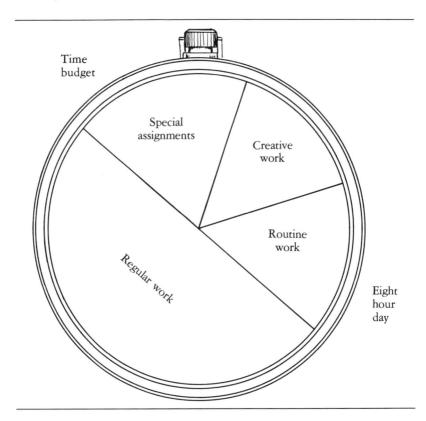

Time budget

Special assignments

Creative work

Routine work

Regular work

Eight hour day

hopping from one job to another. Instead, whenever possible, complete one task before moving to another.

When budgeting your time, the kind or level of work you are doing must be considered as well as the amount of time you will have to spend. The creative things should be done when you are rested, whereas the routine tasks can be done when you are less rested.

IMPROVING PLANNING SKILLS

How can you sharpen your planning skills? The following points should be kept in mind when you devise your plan:

1. Have as complete a knowledge as possible of the patient care that needs to be done.
2. Think clearly and logically, and sort out irrelevant facts.
3. Have a mature sense of values. You must view the plan on your patient-care unit in relation to the hospital's goals, needs, and objectives. To propose a plan that helps your unit to the detriment of another department hinders the hospital's goals.
4. Have foresight. Foresee events that will affect your unit. Holidays, in-service programs, and other such activities will affect the plan.
5. Have a sense of timing. For example, do not leave the stool culture specimen for the evening shift to obtain if the lab closes at 5:00 P.M.
6. Look for training and development needs of staff. Foresee what your staff will need to know in the future, and help them to achieve it. If a patient is about to go to the operating room for a tracheostomy, now is the time to review tracheostomy care with the staff rather than waiting until the patient is back on your unit needing the care immediately.

Once you have devised the plan for the day, utilizing the preceding principles, it should be written clearly, in logical order, and be readily accessible to the staff. The written assignment should be supported by verbal review and clarification; this is the next aspect to be discussed.

How Can the Plan Be Communicated to the Staff?

The nurse who is assigning patient-care tasks to staff members must utilize the management principles of delegation and giving instructions. These two aspects should go hand in hand, for to delegate well means more than entrusting activities to staff. It means defining for each exactly what is to be done. We delegate to relieve our load of detailed responsibilities—in order to have time for other things and, secondly, to develop to the fullest possible extent the potentialities of the staff to whom we have delegated those responsibilities.

GUIDELINES FOR DELEGATION OF TASKS

To get the most from delegation one should proceed with certain guidelines. First, give staff members the proper send-off by specifically outlining what they are to do. Secondly, prepare and support them by indicating confidence in their ability, by giving them reassurance from time to time, and by emphasizing that they may come to you for help whenever they are in doubt. Finally, and most importantly, let them do the job. One of the main principles of modern delegation is that one does not just pass down the work, but that one also passes down to the staff the authority and freedom to handle the details on their own initiative. You may remember having been delegated a job at home such as cooking a meal or cleaning and had your mother give frequent suggestions as to how it could be done. If you felt capable of accomplishing the task alone, you may have been annoyed by the suggestions. Remember how this feels when you are about to interfere with someone else's job.

If the responsibility is new and large or difficult to handle, you may need to check the staff members; but if the staff is well prepared, you may be able to adopt a hands-off policy.

THE NATURE OF DELEGATION

Whenever you delegate, you must be clear in your own mind about the nature of the delegation, because even though a performance is entrusted to another, it is you who retains the ultimate responsibility. You, the leader, are responsible for the care given the patients by your staff members.

When an assignment is a *true* delegation, it has five implicit characteristics:

1. Responsibility is shared with the staff member giving the patient care.
2. Authority is passed along to help the staff member get the job done.
3. Decision-making is shared with or left largely to the staff member.

4. The staff member is given freedom to take actions that that person thinks are needed to reach the objective.
5. The individual accepting the assignment must be held accountable by the delegator.

The leader who perfects the ability to delegate will find it a staff builder because it produces three essential effects: It develops the staff members' sense of responsibility, it enlarges their general understanding, and it increases their job satisfaction.

EFFECTIVE VERSUS INEFFECTIVE DELEGATION

Can you think of units in the hospital in which effective delegation takes place? Can you think of units in which the head nurse holds all the reins of administration and does not delegate enough? As a staff nurse you will find it interesting to watch the return of the head nurse who has been off duty a few days. Some head nurses return with the attitude that the unit must have crumbled in their absence and that they must immediately put it back together again. If in truth things did not run smoothly in the head nurse's absence, the head nurse should start delegating so that the unit can function well in that person's absence. In contrast to this head nurse is the one who returns to the unit calmly after a few days of absence and knows that the staff can function alone. Much more credit is due to this head nurse, who has developed the potential of the staff nurses, than to the one who has been afraid or is unwilling to let go of the reins. The concept of team nursing has been obscured many times because the head nurse has not been able to relinquish to the group leader the authority to lead the staff members. Similarly, leaders who do not delegate well will find themselves flying around trying to do more than they are able to do well.

Delegation can also be carried to the opposite extreme—it can be overdone to the point where the leader relies entirely on the staff. We therefore cannot advocate any cut-and-dry rules in delegation; it remains an art. It should be a reciprocal process in which the delegator instructs the staff and they in turn report on their progress.

REASONS GIVEN FOR FAILURE TO DELEGATE

Managers most frequently give the following reasons for not delegating:

1. The staff members lack experience. I feel insecure about them and am reluctant to take chances.
2. I am too busy to explain things to them.

3. I am afraid their mistakes may harm the patients.
4. I am afraid of losing control.
5. I do not know how to organize my work around others.
6. I like to make all the decisions.
7. The staff members are too busy.
8. I can do it faster and easier myself.

Managers who are guilty of using any of these excuses should reexamine their own performance as leaders, for the ability to work through others is one of the hallmarks of success. Through others one multiplies one's own effectiveness. Managers then use their time to concentrate on those things that bring the greatest return.

EFFECTIVE COMMUNICATION OF PLANS TO STAFF
After you decide what to delegate you need to communicate the plan. C. A. Cerami [1] has made some valuable suggestions as to how to tell others what to do:

1. The simple and routine tasks should be assigned in a direct, straightforward, unapologetic fashion. Do not appear hesitant in your request, but make it clear exactly what you want done and when.
   EFFECTIVE: "Mr. James, I would like you to help Miss Wright ambulate Mr. Gregory and Mr. Williams."
   LESS EFFECTIVE: "Mr. James, I hope you will not mind too much helping Miss Wright, when you have some free time, to ambulate Mr. Gregory and Mr. Williams."
2. Do not confuse the staff with parenthetical thoughts, but keep your statements positive, clear, and courteous.
   EFFECTIVE: "When Mrs. Burn returns from the operating room, please check her urine output, vital signs, dressings, and intravenous fluids every fifteen minutes."
   LESS EFFECTIVE: "When Mrs. Burns returns from the operating room, I guess we had better check her vital signs every thirty minutes, or better yet every fifteen minutes. She may have a Foley catheter; if she does not, try to get her to void. Measure her urine output whether it is a Foley catheter or not. I am not sure what kind of dressing she will have but check it. She might have an intravenous running, but then again it may be discontinued by the time she leaves the recovery room. If she has one, let me know how fast it is running."

3. The assignment should be stated in a manner that will generate a desire to do the job well. In so doing you should convey your interest and enthusiasm for the job, make the job seem important, and convey your confidence that the staff can handle it competently. You may need to "sell" your idea by making it appeal to the other person's point of view.

   EFFECTIVE: "Mr. Shriner is to be ambulated for the first time today. It will be exciting to see how he does for he has really been looking forward to getting out of bed."

   LESS EFFECTIVE: "Mr. Shriner is to be ambulated today. He has been on bed rest two months so he will probably need considerable help."

4. There should be no overlapping of functions. For example, there should be no confusion as to who is to take a patient's blood pressure when he returns from the recovery room.

5. Each staff member should report to one and only one superior; in true team nursing the team member should report to the team leader, not to the head nurse.

6. When you assign jobs, you should indicate when they should be completed, how thoroughly the work should be done, and all the factors involved.

7. Usually some explanation of "why" is necessary in order to spell out precisely what is wanted. If the person receiving the order understands why something is to be done a certain way, or better still, the importance of its being done that way, there is a better chance of its being done correctly. Knowing why will help the staff members use their own judgment along the way. For example, if a nurse told the aide that Mr. Brown was allowed nothing by mouth (NPO) but did not tell her why, the following problem might occur: The aide goes into Mr. Brown's room and removes the water pitcher. He asks why, and all the aide can say is "You are not supposed to have anything to drink." It leaves the patient questioning, and if he wants to know why, the aide has to go back to the nurse to find out the reason for the order. How much more effective it would have been if the nurse had told the aide *why* in the first place!

CHECKING THAT INSTRUCTIONS ARE UNDERSTOOD

It is essential that you check to see that your assignment is understood. You can watch the staff member's face for expressions of doubt or of understanding. Do not ask, "Do you understand?"

because people often reply affirmatively rather than admit that they do not understand. Instead you can ask, "How do you plan to proceed?" or "Can you tell me what steps you are going to take?" or "What are your plans?" The leader can also verify the understanding by checking the progress the staff member is making in completing the assignment.

Sometimes instructions go afoul. The fault may be with the staff member. The staff member may not be listening, may not understand the assignment, or may fail to ask questions to clarify the assignment. The staff member may dislike the person giving the assignment. The simple omission of taking notes may result in an assignment's not being completed properly.

The leader may also be at fault. A *very common* cause of instructions' going afoul is an assumption by the sender that the receiver will understand. Incorrect terminology may be used, however, or the words understood by the sender may not be understood by the receiver. Other possible errors are that the assignment is vague, not positive, or that there is no explanation of why, whereby the receiver does not understand the importance of the assignment. There may be a lack of verification or feedback.

Another common error by the leader is failure to give instructions in a systematic way. The consequences of poor instructions may be that the assignment is not done correctly, completely, or on time; that the patient may be displeased or actually suffer from the lack of assigned care; and that the staff member may also suffer by knowing that the job was not done well. If this should occur, analyze where the breakdown in communication occurred. Once alerted to the possible problems in giving instructions, concentrate on giving them correctly as discussed in this chapter.

What Method of Follow-up Should Be Used?

For further verification that the patient-care assignment is proceeding satisfactorily, the leader uses a method of checking and supervising. The nurse-leader's effectiveness as a first-level supervisor will be measured in terms of the help given the individual staff members. In order to be effective as a helper, the leader must develop a good working relationship with the staff members. This relationship helps meet the needs of the group by providing an atmosphere of security and belonging that precedes job satisfaction.

The staff must view the leader as one skilled in giving patient care. The leader must behave in a manner that is accepted by the group and therefore should become familiar with the expectations of the staff as soon as possible.

CLOSE SUPERVISION

Strauss and Sayles [12] define two types of supervision: *close supervision* and *general supervision*. The *close supervisor* gives the staff member an assignment telling exactly how and in what sequence tasks are to be done. For example, take the case of Mrs. Wagner, the group leader. She is giving Miss Jones, LPN, her morning assignment. "Miss Jones, you are to care for Mr. Smith today. His TPR is to be taken at 7:30 A.M., his blood pressure at 7:45 A.M., his intake and output at 8:00 A.M., complete bath with back care at 8:15 A.M., up in a chair at 8:45 A.M." "He is to ambulate around the room." "Do that before putting him back to bed." "His slippers are in the closet." "He needs to cough deeply every two hours." "Do that after he has ambulated but while he is sitting." And on and on for the remainder of the day. Mrs. Wagner, team leader, does not acknowledge that Miss Jones has any initiative or judgment. Mrs. Wagner then proceeds to check up on Miss Jones frequently to make sure the instructions are being carried out. Miss Jones is not allowed freedom to do her work in her own way. Mrs. Wagner is so busy checking up on the staff members and working alongside them (for she feels she can often do the job better than they can) that her entire day is consumed with short-range problems. One can often find Mrs. Wagner busily performing tasks that could have been delegated to a staff member. Consequently she has no time for training and developing her staff members.

Close supervisors feel the need to hover over staff members to make things come out right. They do not trust their subordinates to do a good job. They are of the school of thought that believes the only way to get a job done is to do it yourself. They may be psychologically insecure.

GENERAL SUPERVISION

In contrast, the *general supervisor* sets goals, tells staff members what is to be accomplished, fixes the limits within which they can work, and lets them decide how to achieve these goals. Instead of rattling off a list of orders, the general supervisor is likely to communicate helpful information or make suggestions. This supervisor explains "why" and points out how the staff's contribution fits into the goals for the day. If Mrs. Wagner were a general supervisor her assignment to Miss Jones might have gone like this: "Miss Jones, you are to care for Mr. Smith today. He had a pneumonectomy done yesterday for cancer of the lung. His vital signs, intake, and output are to be taken every four hours. He needs to be encouraged to cough deeply and to get out of bed to ambulate today to help expand the remaining lung. Our goals for his care are to get him up and about and doing as much as possible for himself in order to use the remaining lung fully, and to prevent development of atelectasis."

General supervisors know that the individual staff members will not perform an assignment in precisely the same way they would, but this does not bother them. They concentrate on objectives and results not details.

General supervisors seek to develop an atmosphere in which staff members feel free to bring their problems to them. The general supervisor has spent time training staff. Therefore, the staff has no need for detailed instruction. The general supervisor thus has time to concentrate on long-range rather than short-range problems.

CHOOSING BETWEEN GENERAL AND CLOSE SUPERVISION
Research [6] has shown that the general supervisor is more productive than the close supervisor. The reason for this is that the general supervisor has time for planning, improving staff relations, and coordinating activities with other departments. The close supervisor, in contrast, is doing the same sort of work as the staff members or may be concentrating on paperwork and short-term activities such as checking up on the staff or arranging for supplies.

Which type of supervisor would be most effective on the patient-care unit? There is some evidence [9] that general supervision is most effective where the job is challenging, where the work cycle is long, and where there is an opportunity for intrinsic job satisfaction. In contrast, where there is little opportunity for creativity and internalized motivation, employees are less likely to perform effectively when left alone. It is important to recognize which staff members find their jobs challenging and satisfying and which ones do not.

Another factor in choosing between close and general supervision is that there are substantial differences in the amount of responsibility people are willing to accept on the job. One person may flourish under supervision that another might find extremely restrictive.

Psychological research [7] provides evidence that the nature of a person's personality affects his attitude toward supervision. Some people have a high need for independence, whereas others prefer to be told what to do. Some employees have become so accustomed to the authoritarian approach in their culture, family, and previous work experience that they regard general supervision as no supervision at all. They may abuse the privilege of general supervision and refuse to accept the responsibilities it demands.

Consider the case of two hospital units supervised by two very different head nurses [3]. The first head nurse (Miss Kelly), though extremely courteous, is very strict with nurses. She insists that conversations be kept to a minimum, and she hands out detailed, unambiguous work assignments to her nurses. The second head nurse (Miss Rogers) has a much more informal, almost chummy relationship with the nurses. She consults with them about problems and changes and has developed a feeling of camaraderie on the floor. Which unit do you think nurses chose to work on? Both units are popular, but to different types of nurses. Some nurses like the security of Miss Kelly's unit where everything goes according to predetermined routine. The staff like having everything structured for them; otherwise they feel lost. They require close guidance. Other nurses prefer Miss Rogers' unit as she allows them independence. They have initiative and self-confidence and respond best when they can assert themselves and work on their own. It is probable that these nurses were permitted more freedom in the home environment and in their study of nursing than were the other nurses. Both types respond better to the style of supervision that fits their life-style.

The overall pattern of supervision is more important than any one aspect of it. A manager who delegates authority but neglects to train the staff to exercise it intelligently may well provide poorer nursing care than the manager who retains all authority.

Both the close and general supervisor must exercise authority. You, the leader, will need to make decisions on your own at times. If your goals are unmet, you must find out who or what was responsible.

RELATIONSHIP OF THE SUPERVISOR WITH STAFF

The supervisor's job is always complicated by the fact that people feel an ambivalence toward authority. People value freedom but may feel lost if they have too much. People like feeling safe, but do not like interference. Most people like to be assured that they are performing well and that they will receive help when needed.

How can leaders exercise authority effectively, but without being restrictive? The kind of working relationship the leaders have, the way they give orders, their fairness, and the way they handle mistakes all affect the way staff members will respond to their authority.

The relationship the leader has with staff members has a lot to do with the way the staff members view their work. They need to feel that their leader approves of their work and of themselves as individuals. The leader can show approval by taking an active interest in staff members, by listening to their problems, by giving praise when it is justified, and by showing tolerance when mistakes are made. The existence of a feeling of approval indicates that the supervisor has demonstrated a personal loyalty to the staff. Because different individuals respond differently to supervision, leaders should adjust their behavior patterns to the staff members' individual personality needs.

Good informal relations on matters that are not directly related to the unit set the stage for better communications between the leader and the staff on problems related to work. Any social barrier will create a communications barrier. If the staff members feel free to talk to the leader about their social life or family problems, they will usually feel free to talk to the leader about problems on the unit. It is the supervisors who set the tone of the relationship, not the staff members. You set the tone by being available. Busy, hurried leaders are going to find staff members reluctant to approach them.

EXCHANGE OF INFORMATION AND IDEAS WITH STAFF
Research indicates that productive supervisors give their staff as much information as possible about what is expected on the unit and what is likely to happen in the future. Referring back to the two different head nurses: Some nurses on Miss Rogers' unit complained because they did not receive enough detailed instructions; and some nurses on Miss Kelly's unit felt insecure because Miss Kelly failed to provide enough information for them to make decisions on their own and had a habit of issuing unexpected and seemingly arbitrary orders.

Encouraging staff members to bring ideas and suggestions to you or to the other staff members also helps foster a healthy working climate.

Another factor in supervision is to avoid playing favorites. It is easy to be unconscious of doing this. You must be fair with all staff members, and if you need to make an exception for one member it should be considered legitimate by all members of the group.

CORRECTING ERRORS OF STAFF MEMBERS

How you handle mistakes is another management skill. You do not want to encourage mistakes, but to insist that mistakes must never be made hampers staff members from assuming any real responsibility. Most nurses make a medication error sometime in their experience. If all medication errors were to be disastrous, either we would have few patients or we would have few nurses left to care for them. Actually, doing something wrong is often the most effective way of learning to do it right. For example, next time the nurse who made the error will read the label more carefully, check the dosage in the *Hospital Formulary*, and read the accompanying literature prior to giving the medication.

If you, the leader, overpunish the staff member who makes a mistake, staff members will avoid any task where a mistake is possible.

If you come into a patient's room and you see the LPN making a mistake, what should you do? If the LPN recognizes her own mistake and takes steps to correct it, then do not criticize. Save your criticism for instances when the staff member is unaware of the mistake or fails to correct the mistake. When a nurse makes a mistake, ask how it happened and then listen to the answer. If the explanation is weak, the nurse will recognize it and so will you. Then ask the nurse to tell you how the mistake can be avoided in the future. You may not agree with the solution, but by using this approach, you encourage staff members to accept responsibility for their actions.

CRITICIZING STAFF ERRORS

Most mistakes are due to ignorance or lack of skill and can be handled through training and without resort to criticism. If negligence is the cause, however, you must let the staff member know you are dissatisfied with the performance. Whyte [13] suggests some rules in offering criticism:

1. The criticism should be voiced in a matter-of-fact manner. Emotionalism will arouse defensive reactions.
2. Criticism should be focused on the error, not on the person.
3. After criticism is stated, it should be dropped, unless the mistake has not been corrected.
4. Criticism should be balanced by giving credit for good work.

How Can the Effectiveness of the Plan Be Evaluated?

The leader looks at the objectives for the day when assessing the plan. These factors can be considered in evaluating the objectives:

1. Did individual staff members complete their assignments on time?
2. Did any staff have excess time? If so, how was this time spent?
3. How did the staff members respond to their assignments? Did they appear to derive satisfaction from the day's work?
4. Were the patients content with the nursing care they received today?
5. Did you, the leader, complete the list of priorities to be accomplished for the day?

In evaluating the plan you may find ways to improve it.

What Alterations May Be Necessary in the Plan?

"The best laid schemes of mice and men often go awry" (Robert Burns). The patient-care unit, unlike the automobile assembly line, is subject to multiple changes. The unit can be besieged by many incidents that result in a change of plans. For example, it is Saturday morning. Two aides call in sick at 6:30 A.M., a patient with a head injury is admitted to the unit from the emergency room at 8:45 A.M., the linen supply is depleted at 9:00 A.M. due to a problem in the linen department, and a cardiac arrest occurs at 1:00 P.M. The leader must be flexible in altering priorities and in changing the plan. Inability to do so threatens the quality of the patient care. As changes are necessary, the leader must once again use the tools for communicating the changes to staff members. The completion of the altered plan must then be followed by an evaluation of its effectiveness.

Group Session

Questions 1–4 are written for group discussion. Get a group of classmates or friends together to discuss these questions if you do not have an opportunity to answer them in a classroom session.

1. Have one or more group members bring to the group the hospital's job descriptions for each level of personnel on the nursing unit. Also bring a description of the staff members and the patients on a given unit on a given day. Have the group work out a day's assignment for each of the staff members assigned to the unit.
2. If you have made assignments on a patient-care unit and have worked an eight-hour shift with this assignment, bring it to the group and discuss your evaluation of the assignment. What changes would you make if you could do it over again?
3. Role play the leader's interaction in the following situations:
   a. The nurse-leader is seeing Mr. Round for the first time. He has been admitted with the diagnosis of emphysema.
   b. The leader is making rounds in the morning and has been told in report that Mrs. Weather is one day postpartum.
   c. The nurse's aide comes to the leader to say that Johnny's mother is sobbing. Johnny is a three-year-old patient with hydrocephalus.
4. A new aide has the following patient to care for: Miss Black, age 28, with nephritis; on an 800 cc fluid restriction per 24 hours; 40 gm protein diet; no salt; accurate intake and output; up to bathroom with help. Role play how you would explain this assignment to the new aide.
5. The work load is heavy today. As you complete the assignments and explain them to the staff, the LPN says angrily, "I cannot possibly do all of that. It is not fair!" How can you, the leader, best handle this situation?
6. Discuss which of the staff members on your unit require close supervision and which ones respond better to general supervision. Under which type of supervision do you work best?
7. As you walk into a four-bed ward, you observe that the orderly has detached the patient's traction ropes to make the bed. What would you do?
8. During the assignment conference you told the aide to turn the patient every two hours. Since then you have been into the patient's room four times, and each time it appeared that the patient was in the same position as the last time you were in the room. What would you say to the aide? If she says she has been too busy to turn him, how would you respond?

Job Description: Nurse's Aide

A. The nurse's aide will be assigned to care for hospitalized patients in all areas of nursing practice except for special care units, including the coronary care unit, the intensive care unit, the recovery room, and the emergency room.
B. The nurse's aide will give basic nursing care as assigned and directed by a registered professional nurse.
C. Functions of nurse's aides include:
   1. Making patients comfortable
   2. Assisting the patients with special needs, such as combing hair
   3. Maintaining a safe and clean environment for the patients
   4. Assisting the patients' families and visitors when needed

    5. Observing patients for specific signs and symptoms directed by the registered nurse

    6. Reporting changes in the patients' behavior or condition to the registered nurse

    7. Assisting other staff members with patient care

D. The nurse's aide may perform the following procedures:

    1. Baths (complete, partial, shower, tub, sitz)

    2. Beds (occupied, unoccupied, postop, and circ-olectric)

    3. Cold applications (ice collar, ice bag, rubber glove)

    4. Pre- and postop care (shock, I & O fractions only, Foley catheter)

    5. Weighing patients

    6. Hematesting stools

    7. Collection of specimens (urine and stool)

    8. Safety measures, such as footboards, bed cradles, siderails, restraints, and posey belts

    9. Ambulating patients

    10. Transferring patients

    11. Admission, transfer, and discharge of patients

    12. Dietary care, including diet forms, giving nourishments, and feeding patients

    13. Giving enemas (soapsuds, tap water, oil retention, Travad, Fleets, or flatus bags)

    14. Taking vital signs, including temperature, pulse, and respiration

CONTROLS

The nurse's aide is ultimately accountable to the head nurse on the unit. The team leader is responsible for making out assignments for the nurse's aide and supervises the care given by the nurse's aide. The nurse's aide is responsible to the team leader for care assigned.

QUALIFICATIONS

The nurse's aide must be a high school graduate who has completed the nurse's aide course given at "X" hospital. The nurse's aide must be a dependable and responsible person who is interested in giving quality nursing care.

References

1. Cerami, C. A.   How to tell others what to do. *Supervision Magazine* Aug. 1955.
2. Dewey, W. E.   You can use your time better. *Factory Management and Maintenance* 111:84–89, Feb. 1953.
3. Hamilton, E.   Delegation. In G. Strauss and L. Sayles, *Personnel: The Human Problems of Management* (3rd ed.). Englewood Cliffs, N.J.: Prentice-Hall, 1972. Pp. 158–159.

4. Kahn, R. L., and Cannell, C. E. *The Dynamics of Interviewing.* New York: Wiley, 1957. Pp. 233–252.

5. Kron, T. *The Management of Patient Care: Putting Leadership Skills to Work* (4th ed.). Philadelphia: Saunders, 1976. Pp. 135–148.

6. Likert, R. *New Patterns of Management.* New York: McGraw-Hill, 1961. Pp. 89–96.

7. McClelland, D. C. *The Achieving Society.* Princeton: Van Nostrand, 1961. Pp. 36–62.

8. Melody, M., and Clark, G. Walking-planning rounds. *Am. J . Nurs.* 67:771–773, April 1967.

9. Morse, N. *Satisfaction in White Collar Jobs.* Ann Arbor: Survey Research Center, University of Michigan, 1953. Pp. 55–67.

10. Richardson, S., Dohrenwend, B., and Klein, D. *Interviewing: Its Forms and Functions.* New York: Basic Books, 1965. Pp. 1–327.

11. Rogers, C. *Client-Centered Therapy: Its Current Practice, Implications and Theory.* Boston: Houghton Mifflin, 1951. Pp. 3–196.

12. Strauss, G., and Sayles, L. *Personnel: The Human Problems of Management* (3rd ed.). Englewood Cliffs, N.J.: Prentice-Hall, 1972. Pp. 139–162.

13. Whyte, W. F. *Leadership on the Work Team* (mimeograph), 1956. Pp. 12–13.

Suggested Reading

Clark, E. L. A model of nurse staffing for effective patient care. *Nurs. Adm.* 7:22, Feb. 1977.

Clark, J. Authority patterns in nursing managent structures. *Nurs. Times* 73:65, May 12, 1977.

Damos, V. R. Management skill: Objectivity. *A.O.R.N.* 25:195, Feb. 1977.

Gellerman, S. W. Supervision: Substance and style. *Harvard Bus. Rev.* 54:89, March/April 1976.

Grant, C. Future trends in health care management. *Ga. Nurs.* 37:2, June 1977.

Hill, B. S. Participative management: A valid alternative to traditional organizational behavior. *Superv. Nurse* 7:19, March 1976.

Holloway, R. C. Management can reverse declining employee work attitudes. *Hospitals* 50:71, Oct. 16, 1976.

La Monica, E., et al. Managerial decision making. *J. Nurs. Adm.* 7:20, May 1977.

Lewis, J. H. Conflict management. *J. Nurs. Adm.* 6:18, Dec. 1976.

Miller, N. How to succeed in nursing management. *Superv. Nurse* 8:18, Oct. 1977.

Munn, H. E., Jr. Measure your nursing supervisor leadership behaviors. *Hosp. Top.* 54:14, Nov./Dec. 1976.

Nelson, M. A. Building a better team. *Nursing '77* 7:65, July 1977.

Pellet, J. Are you making delegation work for you? *A.O.R.N.* 25:865, April 1977.

Stevens, B. J. The delicate art of nursing supervision and leadership. The head nurse as manager. *Nurs. Dig.* 5:13, Fall 1977.

Treat, M., et al. The delicate art of nursing supervision and leadership. The question behind the question. *Nurs. Dig.* 5:1, Fall 1977.

Vance, C. C. How to enrich your management skills. *Nursing '75* 5:65, April 1975.

Veningia, R. Interpersonal feedback: A cost-benefit analysis. *Nurs. Dig.* 5:54, Fall 1977.

Volante, E. M. Mastering the managerial skill of delegation. *Nurs. Dig.* 5:33, Fall 1977.

Watkin, B. Nursing Forum. Do we manage to care? *Nurs. Mirror* 141:48, Oct. 2, 1975.

White, R. Management of the nursing service. *Nurs. Mirror* 143:67, Oct. 28, 1976.

Zorn, J. M. Nursing leadership for the 70s and 80s. *J. Nurs. Adm.* 7:33, Oct. 1977.

10. Appraising Staff Performance

Managers must judge continually the contributions and abilities of the staff members. Certain individuals are more adept at doing one type of work than another, certain ones cannot be depended upon to carry through an assignment to completion, others show great initiative and reliability and can take on projects with a minimum of supervision.

Appraisal of staff performance serves primarily as a training device—to help staff members improve their performance. An effective performance-appraisal program also serves as a rational basis for determining who should be promoted or receive salary increases. It permits staff members on each level to be considered on the same basis as others on the same level. If ratings are linked to promotions, they can serve as a tool for motivation. Performance appraisals need not be limited to identifying those who should be promoted, receive pay increases, or obtain special attention. They can be the springboard for coaching and for helping individuals to set goals for their own development. Employees learn how effective they are and how they can improve and develop.

Performance appraisal is the systematic evaluation of individuals with respect to their performance on the job and their potential for development. Ordinarily the evaluation is made by the individual's immediate superior in the organization, and this is reviewed in turn by that person's superior. Thus, everyone in the organization who rates others is also rated by a superior.

Evaluation Procedures

Health-care agencies should have a well-defined program for the evaluation of personnel. Job descriptions can outline performance standards and should be discussed at the time of employment and again during the employee's orientation to the position. These standards then become the basis for evaluation. It is advisable to have ongoing evaluations at set intervals or whenever the evaluator feels they should be held or when the employee has questions.

A variety of evaluation procedures are used in health-care agencies. The traditional rating form is being replaced in some institutions by a less biased procedure. Various types of evaluation forms will be explained in the following paragraphs.

RATING SCALES

The rating scale is the oldest and most widely used type of rating procedure, and it appears in various forms. Usually the individual doing the rating is given a printed form that contains a number of qualities and characteristics to be rated. This is usually done by the employee's immediate supervisor. An example of this type of form can be found in Appendix A at the end of the chapter.

DRAWBACKS OF TRADITIONAL EVALUATION

The traditional rating scale is subject to certain human errors. One is clarity in standards. Unless all evaluators agree on what terms such as "good" or "excellent" mean, their final ratings simply cannot be compared. For example, the rating scale in one agency includes excellent, very good, fair, satisfactory, and unsatisfactory. One evaluator might describe an aide's performance as very good, whereas another evaluator may describe the same performance as excellent.

A second human error in rating is that people differ in their standards of judgment. Raters may be unaware of their prejudice against staff members whose behavior, attitudes, or values are very different from their own. For example, a head nurse who is always punctual may be prejudiced in evaluating a staff member who usually arrives at work a few minutes late, but who does an excellent job once at work. Having more than one individual rate the employee will reduce the degree of subjectivity. This is exemplified by the Olympic diving championships in which a group of judges rate each contestant.

A third problem is that external considerations may result in easy or hard grading. An evaluator may hesitate to give a low rating to an LPN fearing that ill feelings may develop that will hamper their working relationship. Another evaluator may purposely rate a staff member low the first time in the hope that the next evaluation can be higher and thus show improvement.

A fourth tendency is for the raters to be inclined to give similar ratings on the various points on the evaluation scale. For example, an RN may excel in initiative. The evaluator may then mark additional traits excellent, even though they have not been demonstrated.

A more fundamental criticism of the traditional rating scale is that personality traits rather than measurable objectives are often emphasized. Such traits as learning ability, loyalty, judgment, and enthusiasm are difficult if not impossible to measure. These are personality traits that are difficult to change and whose evaluation is of little value in helping a staff member identify areas for improvement.

NURSE'S DILEMMA IN
EVALUATING STAFF MEMBERS

1. What's the difference between good, excellent, and very good?
2. What's more important — excellent sterile technique or good rapport with patients?
3. If I grade low will he be so offended that our working relationship will suffer?
4. She's very neat, so does this mean she gives thorough nursing care?
5. How can I measure "initiative"?
6. The things that stand out the most in my memory are those that have happened recently.

As a consequence of the foregoing criticisms of traditional rating scales, personnel researchers have developed new rating procedures that are less affected by the raters' personal biases and are less concerned with personality traits. Two well-known forms are forced distribution and the critical incident form.

FORCED DISTRIBUTION RATING
Forced distribution requires the rater to distribute ratings in a pattern to conform with a normal frequency distribution. It uses the same principle as "grading on a curve." Staff members being rated by this technique would be compared to one another. Ordinarily, only one overall rating of ability is given, rather than a series of ratings on separate factors. This form alleviates the tendency to rate all staff members high or low.

This evaluation method also has its shortcomings. The staff members in an agency are a select group of people and do not necessarily have abilities that are distributed according to a normal curve. It is hoped that individuals who would be rated at the low end of the scale in the normal population would not be staff members to begin with.

CRITICAL INCIDENT RATING
The critical incident technique of rating begins with the formulation of critical job requirements or objectives. Once these have been determined, the evaluator looks for critical incidents or examples of the staff member's success or failure to meet the objectives. Schools

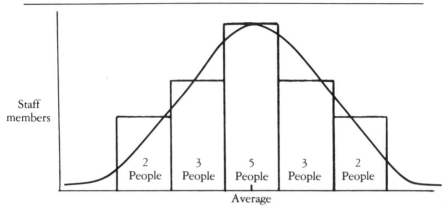

Staff members

2 People | 3 People | 5 People | 3 People | 2 People

Average

Would you evaluate the staff members with the forced distribution method?

of nursing may utilize this method in planning course requirements, employing measurable behavioral objectives as standards for evaluation. Anecdotal notes of clinical experiences serve as examples of the student's ability or inability to meet the objectives.

In order for performance appraisal to be effective for coaching, teaching, and changing undesirable behavior, the staff member needs to know which behaviors are desirable, as well as which ones need improvement. Such incidents will be observed and recorded by the evaluator as they occur.

To keep these data useful, the manager needs to write down what happened or did not happen, the situation in which the action took place, and what was said to the staff member. This information forms a behavioral record, a critical incident report of which the staff member has already been informed and which is now in the staff member's record and is open to review.

The advantage of this rating method is its objectivity, because the anecdotal notes can be evaluated to determine patterns of behavior and progress toward goal achievement that have been going on over a long period of time. Use of the critical incident technique helps the manager who is preparing yearly evaluations from being influenced primarily by what has been observed during the past month. To ensure objectivity the specific incidents to be cited must be recorded promptly. Attempting to remember events that occurred 6 to 12 months earlier without written records would be much less objective. A recent event should not outweigh accumulated evidence. When unfavorable incidents are observed, the evaluator must tell the staff member about it at the time and give the staff member a chance to explain how it occurred. This rating method requires the evaluator to pay close attention to the performance of staff members. The critical incident process compels evaluators to face staff members, a responsibility too many shirk.

When the time comes for the manager to have an evaluation conference with the staff member, the critical incidents will be reviewed. There should be no surprises for the staff member. These specific records are also helpful in cases in which an employee needs to be fired or a student failed.

This technique also serves as a form of coaching. If staff members receive feedback at the time incidents occur, they can be aware of any changes they need to make to improve performance. It will help correct problems before they escalate into larger ones.

When staff members receive continual feedback they can better assess their abilities, which can help them in deciding whether to stay with the current job or seek promotion. The employer too needs to know which employees are ready for increased responsibility and promotion.

FREE-FORM EVALUATION

Another form for evaluation is the free-form essay evaluation record. The free-form essay evaluation does not use scales, checklists, or any other devices. It simply requires the evaluator to write down impressions of the individual. The comments can, if desired by the employer, be grouped under headings.

If done well, this method requires a considerable amount of time from the evaluator. It is also true that the resultant appraisals often depend more upon the skill and effort of the writer-rater than upon the real performance of the people being evaluated.

MANAGEMENT BY OBJECTIVES

Management by objectives is a relatively new approach to performance appraisal that has been designed to overcome some of the problems associated with the traditional appraisal methods. The major elements of management by objectives are as follows:

1. The manager and staff member sit down together at the beginning of the appraisal period to establish measurable goals for the staff member to accomplish. They jointly agree upon and list the principal duties and areas of responsibility of the individual's job.
2. The staff member sets short-term performance goals in coopera-

tion with the manager. The manager guides the process to meet the needs of the patient-care unit.

3. They agree upon criteria for measuring and evaluating performance.

4. They periodically meet to evaluate progress toward the goals. The staff member makes an appraisal of what has been accomplished relative to the targets set earlier. It is substantiated with factual data if possible. The "interview" is an examination by manager and staff member together of the staff member's self-appraisal, and it culminates in a resetting of goals for the next period of time.

5. The manager is supportive through counseling and coaching in helping the staff member achieve the goals.

6. The manager is less the judge and more the helper.

7. The process focuses upon results accomplished and not upon personal traits.

In a nutshell, the manager can say, "What are your plans? How can I help?" At the evaluation interview the manager can ask, "What can you do for the patient unit that I have not given you a chance to do?"

There are many advantages to management by objectives. There is an ever-increasing body of data that clearly shows that when workers are given the opportunity to participate in establishing their own work rules, their performance is significantly improved. By the same criterion, the quality of performance appraisals will be improved if the staff member is given the opportunity to participate in setting work objectives and in evaluating performance against those specific objectives. This procedure would considerably decrease reliance on the single source of information and would tend to reduce the amount of bias.

A sample evaluation form using the principles of management by objectives is in Appendix B at the end of this chapter. This evaluation should include a list of objectives to be met during the coming year, the standards of performance to be met, and major improvements to be made. The items should be specific. For example, in the hospital setting, such a goal for an aide might be: (1) ensure that all patients who are NPO are instructed as to its meaning; (2) place a sign over these patients' beds designating that the patient is NPO. This type of appraisal is consistent with the psychological principle that people work better when they have definite goals that they must meet in specified periods.

A basic requirement for success with this method is that the staff member be interested in the work and in the organization. The individual must have ideas and ambition.

Management by objectives may be difficult to implement in certain cases. The authoritarian manager might find this method difficult to use. The staff member might try to set easily attainable goals in order to meet the objectives. Generally, however, evidence shows that the appraisal-by-results method is superior to traditional appraisal systems.

An experiment contrasting the goals method to the rating scale was conducted by Morton, Rothaus, and Hanson [4]. First the subordinates were rated by the standard trait-rating scale. Then both the subordinates and superiors reported their feelings and experiences on a behavior-rating scale. Finally, the superiors and subordinates jointly participated in the goal method and again reported their feelings and experiences on a behavior-rating scale. The results showed that with the goal approach there was greater agreement between the supervisor and subordinate. There was also less resistance to suggestions, a friendlier attitude, a greater sense of responsibility by the subordinates regarding the area in which change was needed, a clearer view of the routes to improvement, and greater eagerness to change.

Management by objectives differs from traditional rating methods in that it shifts the emphasis from appraisal to analysis. The subordinates are examining themselves in order to define not only their weaknesses but also their strengths and potentials. One of the main differences of this approach is that it rests on the assumption that individuals know—or can learn—more than anyone else about their own capabilities, needs, strengths, weaknesses, and goals. The conventional approach, on the other hand, makes the assumption that the superior can know enough about subordinates to decide what is best for them.

The proper role for the manager is to listen and advise, guide, and encourage staff members to develop their own potentials, which will (1) lead to increased knowledge and skill, (2) contribute to organizational objectives, and (3) test staff members' appraisals of themselves. The knowledge and active participation of both manager and staff member are necessary components of this approach.

PEER REVIEW

As health-care professionals, nurses collectively monitor and evaluate the health care they provide, thus assuring quality care. Peer review is an essential component of quality assurance. The American

Nurses' Association [1] has written that peer review occurs when those people who deliver a specific type of care develop norms, standards, and criteria for review and carry out the review process for members of their own profession.

Peer review is currently being implemented in some schools of nursing and health-care agencies. Registered nurses with the same role expectation or job description or both are examining the nursing care given by their peers. Thus, operating room nurses give peer reviews to operating room nurses, and delivery room nurses review performances of other delivery room nurses.

The purpose of peer review is to measure the quality of care being given patients, to build on the strengths of the nurses being reviewed, and to identify the nurses' deficiencies or limitations to assist them in improving the quality of patient care given. The results of the peer review may be used in determining advancements and salary increases.

Peer review is based on nursing standards. If peer review were to be implemented on an obstetrical unit, for example, the first step to be taken would be to identify the quality of care to be given an obstetrical patient. The nurses being reviewed would be evaluated on their ability to give the quality of patient care defined by the standards or objectives. These standards or objectives are observable and measurable.

An example of how peer review could be implemented is as follows: The nurses on a 35-bed postpartum unit were chosen to initiate peer review on a trial basis. This unit was selected because of its high standards of care, the cohesiveness and maturity of its staff, and the willingness of its staff to cooperate in the trial study. Whenever a change is to be initiated on a trial basis, it is helpful to start on a unit that has the greatest potential for success. The nurses were given time to discuss the implications of the change and what it would mean to them personally and professionally. The RNs on the unit researched and wrote out the standards of care to be given the postpartum patient. Twelve RNs were to be part of the peer review. Each RN had the opportunity to review and evaluate the performance of at least one peer and to be evaluated by two or three peers. The emphasis was on objectively judging the quality of patient care given, not on finding fault with the nurse.

The nurses had mixed feelings about the peer review, both desiring knowledge of how they could improve yet feeling defensive about their shortcomings being identified by their peers. Because the

12 nurses involved respected their colleagues, apprehension was kept to a minimum. The nurses doing the review had scrutinized the practice of the nurse they reviewed. Therefore, they were able to compliment the nurse on accomplishments as well as make suggestions on how to improve. It became a learning experience for both the reviewers and the nurses being reviewed.

Peer review is possible when nurses have trusting relationships and can work together to set standards for which they are accountable. Under this system nurses can continually grow and develop professionally to improve patient care.

Evaluation Conferences

In order for evaluations to be a tool for staff development, they must be shared with the staff members concerned. Some agencies have the manager hold evaluation conferences with new staff members at the conclusion of their third and sixth months on the job and yearly thereafter. Oftentimes, however, the evaluation conference is allowed to fall by the wayside. One head nurse told the author that she had never received an evaluation as a staff nurse, and therefore did not know how to evaluate the staff members.

Evaluation conferences give staff members a source of feedback about performance on the job and provide the opportunity for the manager to counsel staff members on ways to improve performance.

In addition to performance-appraisal discussions, interviews may be held for such purposes as correcting mistakes, gauging reactions to orders, settling disputes between employees, and helping resolve personal problems that affect performance on the job. Other important purposes are discipline and grievance handling.

DIRECTIVE AND NONDIRECTIVE INTERVIEWS

In the *directive interview* the manager keeps the initiative and controls the conversation. The manager starts with a set of assumptions, asks direct questions to support or modify these assumptions, and then reaches a decision based upon them and whatever added information is gained from the questions. The directive interview has several disadvantages. Staff members may be put on the defensive or may say only what they think the manager wants to hear. It usually fails to reveal the staff member's true feelings.

The *nondirective interview,* sometimes called the *counseling inter-*

view, is a much preferred method for getting staff members to
express themselves freely, for improving understanding between
people, and for working out solutions to problems. The principles
and practices of nondirective interviewing were developed in the
Hawthorne research at the Western Electric Company and by Carl
Rogers and his followers [6, 7].

The four stages in the nondirective interview process are:

1. Development of rapport
2. Expression of feelings
3. Development of facts
4. Discovery of solutions

The manager adopts a friendly, patient, understanding attitude and
tries to put the person at ease and to establish a feeling of rapport.
Their past relationship determines in large part whether the individual feels free to speak openly.

The nondirective interview is essentially a listening one. Neutral
rather than pointed questions are asked. Try to draw the other
person out and refrain from moralizing, preaching, or admonishing.

After feelings have been expressed and understood by both, the
next stage is to develop relevant factual information. The manager
can ask such questions as "How did the difficulty arise?", "Can you
tell me more about that aspect?", or "Why do you think it happened
that way?"

Solutions to problems can evolve in many ways. Sometimes listening to and supporting staff members is enough to help them work
out their own solutions. The manager may need to make suggestions
but should avoid "masterminding" the solution.

DIFFICULTIES IN GIVING EVALUATION INTERVIEWS
Evaluation interviews are not easy. Most people have mixed feelings
about being evaluated, both resenting it and seeking it out. They
desire feedback on "where they stand," and yet assessment is a threat
to independence and autonomy. Staff members often hope their
strengths will be recognized and their weaknesses overlooked. Evidence suggests that staff members tend to rate their own performance higher than do their evaluators; consequently, the interview
can be a deflating experience [3].

The informative and motivational purposes of appraisal cannot be
served unless the staff member being evaluated desires and ap-

preciates constructive criticism. Substantial controversy exists as to whether staff members in fact want to know of their shortcomings. It is the position of the authors that if the criticism is timely, skillfully offered, and related to jointly determined standards, friction will not necessarily be the final result.

Most managers endorse performance appraisal in principle, but few would initiate an evaluation program on their own. Personnel specialists [3, 5] report that most managers carry out performance-appraisal interviews only when strong control procedures are established to ensure that they do.

Managers may be uncertain as to the consequences of negative appraisals. Most managers fear that negative appraisals, or even negative portions of an otherwise favorable appraisal, will discourage staff members rather than serve to motivate. If, as is usually the case, managers do most of the talking during the interview, then they are not doing much listening. If they are not listening, then they are not gaining any insight into staff members' problems.

Some managers "forget" about evaluation interviews. Others hand staff members the form in an embarrassed fashion without asking for comments or replies from the staff member. Even managers who understand principles of supervisory development feel uncomfortable when they have to criticize staff members. If the evaluation form is the traditional type, the manager may hesitate to "judge" the staff member or to "play God." People feel guilty when they criticize others and therefore fear appraising honestly. To avoid ill feeling, many evaluators avoid unpleasant truths. The result is an evaluation in name only.

Fortunately, there are group methods for relieving guilt and for helping managers understand the value of accurate evaluations. One method is to have a group of nurses at the same peer level discuss their problems in giving appraisals. In-service education could also set up a specific program as outlined by Levinson [2]:

1. Group discussion among peers concerning their feelings about appraising subordinates
2. Group discussion resulting in advice from each other on the specific problems that each anticipates in appraising individuals
3. Role playing appraisal interviews
4. Actual appraisals
5. Group discussion to review the appraisals, problems encountered, both anticipated and unanticipated, lessons learned, and skill needs that may have surfaced

GUIDELINES FOR EVALUATION INTERVIEWS

Some guidelines will be given for the nurse giving an evaluation interview or conference. In preparing for the evaluation, remind staff members of the time so that they too can prepare for it. Prior to the interview, they should have a copy of the form that is used and review their job description and any targets or goals that they are attempting to meet. If they have had an evaluation before, review what was written and refresh in your mind what has been discussed previously. Consider what questions they might have about such things as opportunity for promotion. Think of what you have done to help or hinder their development.

Decide what the goal is for the interview. You will probably want to stimulate them to greater effort, help them understand where improved performance is needed, let them know how effective they are, and help them work out specific steps for their own improvement and development.

Plan what you are going to say. The primary emphasis should be on helping them to improve their work results. In so doing you can explore why better results were not obtained in certain areas, in what respect improvement is needed, and what the employees might do to get better results in the future. In planning what you say, try to put yourself in their shoes and think what your reaction would be if these things were said to you.

Plan to tell them what they are doing well, but also ask them about the things that they are not doing especially well. Frequently they will know best what their shortcomings are. Do not dwell on past errors if you discussed them at the time they occurred (as you should have). Have specific suggestions for methods of improvement. Remember that you are evaluating the work, not the person. Avoid words that sound critical or antagonistic, such as "faults," "mistakes," and "illogical." Do not compare them to other staff members.

It is important for the evaluator to have a helpful attitude—not the attitude of a judge or a superior talking down to an inferior. You can ask yourself:

1. Do I feel genuinely friendly to the staff members?
2. Am I interested in them?
3. How can I be helpful to them?
4. How can I encourage them to express themselves?
5. I may be wrong. Can I admit it?
6. How can I express the evaluation so that they will try to do better?

7. Am I thinking of my feelings more than their feelings?
8. If we disagree, will I argue?

Allow a private, comfortable setting for the interview. You should have ample time set aside free from interruptions. Make the staff members comfortable and begin by stating the purpose of the interview and by assuring them that you want to get their views.

The secret of success is putting yourself in the staff members' place and seeing things from their point of view. Do not jump to conclusions or assume you understand, but get them to express their thoughts and ideas. Refrain from dominating the discussion with your own ideas. Let them talk, and as they do, be a good listener. Avoid talking about your own experiences.

During the discussion amplify points with specific facts and occurrences. For example, the statement "Uses good judgment" should be expanded with examples such as "Notified the module leader promptly when patient's urine output suddenly decreased." Give credit for accomplishments, and review goals not accomplished or areas in which improvement is needed. Explore why and how. Notice what they do not say.

Some questions that are helpful to ask the person you are evaluating are:

1. Are aspects of your job defined adequately?
2. Are you challenged?
3. Do you feel your work is appreciated?
4. Do you feel supported?
5. Are you informed and consulted when necessary?
6. Do you have opportunities to use your initiative?

SOME PROBLEMS THE EVALUATOR MAY ENCOUNTER
Occasionally the interview runs into snags. Sometimes you find that staff members will not open up. They answer direct questions briefly but do not enter into the conversation freely. You do not know if they are nervous, angry, or if this is their nature. You can try to discuss something other than the evaluation just to get them to talk. Once they begin talking, they may then talk about the evaluation. Show a special interest in what they say.

Occasionally the persons being evaluated become angry even though you have been tactful. If this should occur, be a good listener as they may be expressing feelings of insecurity, disappointment, or resentment. When they calm down, be sure they understand you will not hold this against them. Go out of your way to be friendly to them in the next few days.

Another problem in interviewing is the employees' agreeing too quickly with everything you say. It may be that they do not understand, but more frequently they want to avoid criticism. Be sure to emphasize strongly the areas that need improvement and outline how you intend to follow up on these plans.

Long-term employees need special treatment. They often need reassurance, and their pride may suffer when they are being evaluated by a younger person. They will probably be highly appreciative of recognition of their judgment and skill.

In closing the interview, review the points on which you have agreed and encourage the staff members to come to you if they have questions or suggestions. The evaluator has the responsibility to follow through to see that staff members are achieving the goals discussed.

OUTLINE OF EVALUATION INTERVIEW
The following outline is an example of how an interview could be conducted:

1. The head nurse tells staff members the purpose of the interview and that it is designed to help them do a better job.
2. The head nurse presents the evaluation, giving the strong points first and then the weak points.
3. The head nurse asks for comments on the evaluation, anticipating that defensive or hostile feelings may be expressed about the negative points. Staff members are allowed to blow off steam. Resenting what is said, defending oneself, or "putting them in their place" gets the evaluator emotionally involved and may stop people from expressing their feelings. Find out why staff members do not agree instead of trying to prove they are wrong.
4. The head nurse asks staff members to discuss the progress they are making, what areas need improvement, and methods for improvement.
5. The interview concludes with the head nurse and staff members discussing the direction for improvement. Both how the staff members can improve and how the head nurse can assist are discussed.

PROVIDING OPPORTUNITIES FOR STAFF MEMBERS
TO EXPRESS VIEWPOINTS

The manager should accept any criticism from staff members without argument. If this is poorly handled, the conference can lead to hostility rather than understanding.

Some managers start the interview with "Tell me how you think you are doing." This has the advantage of letting the staff members express their viewpoints first. Some individuals would rather point out their weaknesses to the manager than have the manager point them out. Others, however, feel that they do not want to expose their opinions until after they have read what their manager has written.

VARYING OBJECTIVES ACCORDING TO THE INDIVIDUAL

The objectives of the interview vary from one person to another. For example:

1. If a weakness is difficult to correct, such as shyness in an aide, or a speech difficulty in an LPN, there is no point in discussing it at all.
2. If the weaknesses are correctable, it is often better to wait for staff members to bring them up when they see fit.
3. If performance is so unacceptable that staff members may be discharged, they should receive a warning. To be genuinely helpful you should face the problem at the earliest possible date, while there is some hope of helping the employees.
4. If employees have done an outstanding job, you may want to help these individuals use their abilities to fullest advantage. This may result in a better job.
5. If employees have not improved, it is best to be frank and direct as to whether they are in the right job. Some nurses may really dislike nursing but have yet to face up to the fact. They might be much more successful at a different job.
6. If employees are just sliding by, it is helpful to find out how they feel about their job. Are they happy in their work?

Performance Appraised: Conclusions

In conclusion, the primary objective of performance appraisal is to encourage and support development of an employee toward meeting the objectives of the institution. Providing for evaluation of employees at all levels emphasizes the expectations of everyone to progress in position, be it at the top, bottom, or middle of the organizational chart. To progress rather than regress, an organization must help motivate its personnel to continuous development. This substantiates the need to comment on weaknesses when they exist; to avoid this denies the purpose of performance appraisal. For criticism to be beneficial, however, it must be accompanied by constructive suggestions for improvement. The likelihood of keeping the evaluation objective will be enhanced if the evaluator's goal is to help the employee rather than to justify the appraisal. There must be leveling, honesty, and helpfulness.

The advantages of a systematic appraisal system to the health-care agency are that: (1) employee strengths and weaknesses can be routinely assessed, (2) it can provide evidence to terminate employees who have had unsatisfactory achievement, (3) it can reveal areas of need for in-service education, and (4) it can serve as periodic feedback to employees.

Study Questions

Questions 1 and 2 are written for group discussion. Get a group of classmates or friends together to discuss these if you do not have a classroom opportunity for discussing them.

1. Miss Walker, RN, age 22, started working on your unit three months ago. She is an extremely enthusiastic worker with lots of good ideas. As a leader, she is short on patience with the staff members. She is constantly pushing them and is annoyed when she finds them taking a break. The staff morale suffers when Miss Walker is leader. During conferences, she has excellent suggestions, but she dominates the discussion. You are concerned about the animosity developing between her and some other staff members. As a head nurse this is the first evaluation you have given Miss Walker.

   a. What should your strategy be in handling the evaluation interview with Miss Walker?

   b. Role play this interview. Miss Walker is sure her ideas are good, and she is pressing for a head-nurse position in the hospital.

2. Miss Saunders, age 25, is an LPN. She is best described as dumpy, quiet, and withdrawn. She often asks the team leader questions that she should be able to answer for herself, given her LPN background. Miss Saunders lacks initiative and needs detailed instructions. Team members ignore her, and she is a loner. Self-confidence appears to be lacking in Miss Saunders. She never says a word in a team conference unless asked a question directly, and then the answer is brief. How would you interview Miss Saunders for her three-month review?

   a. What will be your strategy?

   b. Role play this interview. Miss Saunders responds minimally during the interview.
3. What evaluations did you find most helpful in nursing school? Did any serve as a motivation for change? Which were least helpful? Why?
4. What were your feelings prior to an evaluation conference, during the conference, and after the conference when you were the one being evaluated?
5. Which staff members would you be most reluctant to evaluate in a conference? Why? Which person would be easiest to evaluate? Why?
6. Is it possible for individuals to identify for themselves areas of weakness and areas of strength?

Appendix A
Evaluation Form for Nurses' Aide

Place a check mark in the appropriate column; comments may be added

	Excellent	Very Good	Average	Poor	Unsatisfactory	Comment
	A	B	C	D	E	
1. Technical Skills						
a. Quality of work (Performs procedure correctly, completely)						
b. Quantity of work (Finishes assignments adequately)						
c. Ability to observe (Makes thorough observations of patients)						
d. Emotional support to patients (Recognizes patient needs and acts accordingly)						
e. Reports (Reports accurately, thoroughly, promptly)						
f. Practice of safety (Observes safety in care of patients and equipment)						
2. Group Member						
a. Follows instructions						
b. Cooperates with staff members						
c. Communications (Communicates effectively with patients, visitors)						
d. Contributions (Makes suggestions for improving patient care)						
3. Attitudes						
a. Adaptability (Accepts change; adjusts smoothly)						
b. Etiquette (Is polite, thoughtful, and kind)						
c. Responsibility (Is responsible for work; is concerned for welfare of others)						
d. Initiative (Sees tasks to be done; volunteers)						
e. Supervision (Willingly accepts directions, assignments, constructive criticism)						
f. Interest (Asks questions; appears to enjoy work)						
g. Self-improvement (Tries to improve)						
h. Learning ability (Learns easily)						
4. Personal Hygiene						
a. Is neat, clean, and well groomed						
5. Attendance						
a. Reports on duty promptly; no excessive absences						

Appendix B
Performance Appraisal

The person being evaluated and the evaluator should prepare for the evaluation conference by individually completing the following form. The conference should include a review of both persons' expectations, and the discussion should focus on determination of realistic objectives and standards for the work of the person being evaluated. Each person should keep a copy of the corrected form. This can then be used to check progress during the year and to compare accomplishments with the objectives at the end of the year.

Objectives for the Year. (Determine goals for work to be accomplished and list them in an order of priority.)

Standards. (Outline specific plans for what ought to be achieved during the year. Include information about materials, supplies, human resources, and assistance needed to achieve the objectives stated above. Standards should incorporate quality as well as quantity statements to facilitate measurement.)

Plan for Personal Growth. (Outline specific plans you have for improving your abilities, knowledge, and skills. This can include formal and informal educational plans as well as personal objectives for improving the effectiveness of your performance.)

Year-End Evaluation. (Compare objectives with actual accomplishments. Identify reasons for differences in results, and determine how the desired results can be obtained in the future. Again, both the person being evaluated and the evaluator should prepare their thoughts individually in advance of the conference.)

Objectives Achieved

Objectives Not Achieved: Analysis of Reasons and
Plan for Future Improvement

Results of Plan for Personal Growth: Plans for the Future

References

1. American Nurses' Association. Philosophy of Peer Review, Peer Review Guidelines (pamphlet). American Nurses' Association, Nov. 1973.
2. Levinson, H.   Appraisal of what performance? *Harvard Bus. Rev.* 54:44, July/August 1976.
3. Meyer, H. H., Kay, E., and French, J. P. P., Jr.   Split roles in performance appraisal. *Harvard Bus. Rev.* 23:123, 126, Jan./Feb. 1965.
4. Morton, R. B., Rothaus, P., and Hanson, P. C.   An experiment in

performance appraisal and review, *J. Am. Soc. Train. Direct.* 15:19, May 1961.
5. Parker, J. W., Taylor, E. K., Barrett, R. S., and Martens, L.   Rating scale content: Relationship between supervisory and self-ratings. *Pers. Psych.* 12:49, 1959.
6. Roethlisberger, F. J., and Dickson, W. J.   *Management and the Worker.* Cambridge, Mass.: Harvard University Press, 1939. Pp. 270–291.
7. Rogers, C. R.   *Counseling and Psychotherapy.* Boston: Houghton Mifflin, 1942. Pp. 115–128.

Suggested Reading

Cain, C., and Luchsinger, V.   Management by objectives: Applications to nursing. *J. Nurs. Adm.* 8:35, Jan. 1978.
Carroll, S. J., Jr., and Tosi, H., Jr.   *Management by Objectives.* New York: Macmillan, 1973.
Dau, G. J.   The appraisal process. *Superv. Nurse* 7:39, Aug. 1976.
Fleishman, E. A.   *Studies in Personnel and Industrial Psychology* (rev. ed.). Homewood, Ill.: Dorsey Press, 1967. Section 2.
Haar, L. P., et al.   Performance appraisal: Derivation of effective assessment tool. *Nurs. Dig.* 5:38, Fall 1977.
Hamric, A. B., Gresham, M. L., and Eccard, M.   Staff evaluation of clinical leaders. *J. Nurs. Adm.* 8:18, Jan. 1978.
Humble, J.   *Management by Objectives in Action.* New York: McGraw-Hill, 1970.
Kellogg, M. S.   *Closing the Performance Gap.* New York: American Management Association, 1967.
Koontz, Harold.   *Appraising Managers As Managers.* New York: McGraw-Hill, 1971.
Lasagna, J. R.   Make your MBO pragmatic. *Harvard Bus. Rev.* 49:64–68, Nov./Dec. 1971.
Levinson, H.   Appraisal of what performance? *Harvard Bus. Rev.* 54:30, July/Aug. 1976.
McGregor, D.   An uneasy look at performance appraisal. *Harvard Bus. Rev.* 50:133, Sept./Oct. 1972.
Meyer, H. H., Kay, E., and French, J. P. P., Jr.   Split roles in performance appraisal. *Harvard Bus. Rev.* 23:123, Jan./Feb. 1965.
Oberg, W.   Make performance appraisal relevant. *Harvard Bus. Rev.* 50:61, Jan./Feb. 1972.
Odiorne, G. S.   Management by objectives: Antidote to future shock. *Nurs. Adm.* 5:27, Feb. 1975.
Patz, A. L.   Performance appraisal: Useful but still resisted. *Harv. Bus. Rev.* 51:74, May/June 1973.
Rieder, G. A.   Performance review—a mixed bag. *Harvard Bus. Rev.* 51:61, July/Aug. 1973.
South, J. C.   The performance profile: A technique for using appraisals effectively. *J. Nurs. Adm.* 8:27, Jan. 1978.
Stevens, B. J.   Performance appraisal: What the nurse executive expects from it. *Nurs. Dig.* 5:48, Fall 1977.

11. Discipline

Discipline is necessary to all organized working units. The staff members must control their individual urges and cooperate for the common good of the health-care agency. Individual employees need to conform to the code of behavior established by the agency administration.

Skill in achieving discipline in the work place is an important qualification for a manager. Leaders also need this skill in working with staff members.

Positive discipline involves creation of an attitude whereby staff members conform willingly to the agency's established rules and regulations. It is achieved when the nurse-manager applies principles of positive motivation, when sound leadership is exercised by supervision, and when the entire agency is managed efficiently. The staff members, both as individuals and as a group, adhere to the desired standards of behavior because they understand, believe in, and support them.

Self-Discipline

The best discipline, of course, is self-discipline. Most people want to do a good job and do their share by the rules established. Once people understand what is expected of them, they generally can be counted on to do their job correctly.

If the rules established are viewed by the staff members as fair, they will generally observe them without question. They obey the rules because the rules are reasonable, rather than because they fear punishment. Rules such as coming to work on time, carrying out patient-care assignments, reporting to the nurse-leader, and not stealing agency supplies are viewed by staff members as reasonable and a necessary condition of work.

Group Norms and Discipline

A norm is a group-established standard of expected behavior. People do not behave as isolated, independent individuals. Instead, their behavior is strongly conditioned by the pressures, norms, and culture of the groups to which they belong. The social groups on a work unit frequently exercise very strong control over the behavior of their individual members. These group-established standards of behavior are not written down, but are often expressed orally. The group enforces its standards by social pressure.

Most work groups exercise a stabilizing effect upon the conduct of their members. If the nurse-manager has good relations with the staff members and if the staff members respect the rules of conduct established by the nurse-manager, then this group discipline works in support of management's objectives. The successful manager is one who understands the nature of group forces, who is perceptive to group action, and who can blend group goals with those of the organization.

If the nurse-manager has built a cohesive, loyal work group, then its members will adhere generally to the manager's disciplinary efforts. The nurse-manager can lead discussions covering agency rules and regulations, as well as the need for them. The staff members can discuss how these rules apply to them in their own work situation. If the group as a group understands and believes in the rules, it will often exert social pressure upon its members to ensure that they live up to them. This also applies to unofficial rules and standards accepted by the group. For example, one patient-care unit has an unwritten agreement that any staff member is to answer any patient's light. For a staff member to say, "That isn't my patient," and not answer a patient's light is unacceptable to the group.

Most staff members are tolerant of an occasional infraction of their written and unwritten rules. If Mrs. Jones had a late night celebrating her tenth wedding anniversary and is slow on the job the next day, this can be overlooked if she does her part the rest of the time. But staff members resent seeing someone else "get away with murder" while they are doing a full day's work. As one nurse's aide said, "We're all here to do our job. It really bugs me when I'm working hard and the other aides are goofing off in the lounge while I'm answering all the patients' lights." Lax performance by some may result in lowering the level of performance by all. Thus, enforcing the rules strengthens the group's informal efforts at correction.

Responsibility of the Nurse-Manager
COMMUNICATING RULES
What is the nurse-manager's responsibility in ensuring good discipline? All rules and policies should be communicated to the staff

members. A new staff member should receive information concerning agency policy in a written pamphlet and in an orientation session. In orienting a new person, expected work performance should be explained, as well as what help is available in achieving it. New rules or policy should be communicated to staff members in a written memo to be placed on the bulletin board or added to their policy book. It helps if someone can explain the reason for and background of the policy to the staff members. Before you penalize staff members they must know the rules they are accused of having violated. The rules introduced should seem reasonable to the staff members if they are expected to be followed. For example, a policy stating that all requests for vacations must be submitted one year in advance would seem quite unreasonable. Such a policy might breed "hate and discontent."

FIRM ENFORCEMENT

Rules and policies serve to draw the lines of limitations and freedom for staff members. Therefore, rules must be enforced firmly and fairly. L. Cassels [3] writes that the average worker's natural inclination to obey the rules can be dissipated by lax or inept enforcement policies. Staff members can develop contempt for nurse-managers who allow regulations to be disregarded. Numerous attitude surveys have shown that staff morale is highest in organizations whose members are conscious of being held to a high standard of performance. Reflect for a moment. Would you be happiest working with a nurse-manager who is firm but fair in expecting staff members to give high quality of patient care; or, in contrast, with one whose standards and leadership are lax and staff members do as they please when they please? To achieve constructive discipline, the manager must set a good example.

FAIR ENFORCEMENT

Rules need to be enforced fairly. Is it fair to reprimand an aide for arriving at work 30 minutes late while ignoring the fact that an RN is also 30 minutes late? The rules should apply to everyone and be enforced 24 hours a day, seven days a week. Consistency of treatment is an important principle and one that is easily ignored. Inconsistency can occur because managers in different areas have different standards of what they expect and different tolerance levels when staff members deviate from the standards.

The best way to achieve consistency of treatment and application of the rules is through supervisory training courses and by consistent action by higher management on a day-to-day basis as cases are brought up.

The need for consistency does not mean that two persons committing an identical offense must always receive identical penalties. The background and circumstances of each case may call for differential treatment. But consistency does require that both employees know that they have violated a rule. You must not condone the infraction by one and not the other, but the punishment should fit the offender as well as the offense. If the aide mentioned previously has been 30 minutes late six times in one month and this was the first time the RN was late, genuine fairness requires that each be treated differently. The RN needs to be corrected but does not deserve a harsh punishment.

The basic aim of disciplinary action is to encourage adherence to the rules in the future rather than to punish passing infractions.

Types of Penalties

What are the penalties for wrongdoings? Obviously, penalties must be tied to the gravity of the offense. Some offenses require immediate and final discipline (such as stealing or drug abuse). Many organizations have a progressive system; this means that there is a sequence of penalties from less severe to more severe. Ordinarily it includes these steps outlined by G. Strauss and L. Sayles [5]: (1) oral warning, (2) written warning, (3) disciplinary layoff, and (4) discharge.

The oral warning is given according to the principle presented in a previous chapter about correcting an error promptly. If the aide is 30 minutes late to work, she should be corrected promptly—not six months later during an evaluation conference. The written warning is psychologically more severe than the oral warning since it goes in the employee's record.

Disciplinary layoffs are next in severity. The employee is sent home for several days or weeks without pay. Discharge is the most severe penalty. It is hard not only on the employee, but also on the organization. An RN who is fired must look for a new job and may have difficulty gaining employment. The agency too suffers, for it must hire and orient someone to replace the RN.

Avoiding Resentment

Enforcing discipline puts you, the nurse-manager, in a difficult position. You work with the staff members on a daily basis and want to be regarded as a source of help. Disciplining a staff member is painful for you as well as for the staff member. How can you do it without generating resentment? When you reprimand a staff member, tell (1) what was done that was wrong, (2) why it was wrong (the rule that was violated), and (3) what will happen if it is done again. Then quickly, while it is still fresh in your mind, write a memo on how you handled the situation and what you told the staff member. The written memo becomes part of the staff member's performance record.

The "Hot Stove" Rule

An old but well tested rule for discipline called the "hot stove" rule was advocated by Douglas McGregor [5]. His rule says that when you touch a hot stove, you are burned:

1. Immediately (Your hand gets burned as soon as you touch the stove.)
2. With warning (You knew what would happen if you touched it.)
3. Impersonally (It burned you because you touched it, not because it was you.)
4. Consistently (If your neighbor touched it, it would burn him too.)

The hot stove discipline emphasizes that the act was wrong—not the person.

Let us look at what happens when the principles for discipline are not followed:

Mrs. Slow, RN, has a bad tardiness record. She comes in 30 minutes late but thinks the head nurse is too busy to notice. The head nurse says nothing. By noon, Mrs. Slow assumes that she will not be reprimanded. At 3:15 P.M. the head nurse explains to Mrs. Slow that she has filed a written warning that will be put in her record.

Mrs. Slow is angry with the head nurse and the discipline. She feels that the head nurse was pretending not to notice the offenses until enough were gathered to result in disciplinary action. If the head nurse had followed the hot stove rule, the discipline would have been *immediate* and Mrs. Slow would have seen the act of tardiness disciplined rather than experiencing the discipline as a personal affront.

In order to maintain discipline in the work place, the staff members need to understand what offenses will lead to discipline and what the discipline will be if the offense occurs. For example, a policy states that 30 minutes will be allowed for lunch. The manager has not enforced it, and some staff members take 30 minutes for lunch one day and 40 minutes another day. No one expects the manager to rigidly enforce the rule since it has not been enforced in the past. If the manager were to suddenly choose a staff member to punish for infraction of the rule, it would be without warning. If the manager wanted the rule enforced, the better method would be to announce that infringements would not be tolerated. This would serve as the *warning*. The nurse would also need to explain what disciplinary action would result if an infraction of the rule occurred.

If on Monday you require staff members to ambulate patients at least twice during the day, you should be *consistent* and expect the same performance on Tuesday unless extenuating circumstances intervene. You must also remember consistency when you would rather overlook disciplining some rule breaker. This aspect of consistency is hard to maintain; it means not playing favorites by disciplining some and not disciplining others.

Impersonality is another rule. C. Argyris [2] states that discipline is most effective and has the least negative effects on individuals if the individual feels that the behavior at the particular moment is the only thing being criticized and not the total personality.

The Disciplinary Action

When disciplinary action becomes necessary, attempt to keep communication lines open. You want to learn the basic reason for the incorrect behavior, not the excuse for it.

Incorrect: RN: Miss Watkins, according to Mr. Write you have not been into his room for three hours. Didn't I tell you yesterday that he needs hourly measurements of intake and output and needs turning every two hours?
Correct: RN: Miss Watkins, Mr. Write tells me you haven't been in to check him for three hours. Can you tell me why?

Once you decide what discipline is appropriate, impose it quietly, impersonally, and in private.

Once you have disciplined a staff member, there is a natural tendency to avoid or to act differently toward the individual. Make a conscious effort not to do either of these, as your relationship with the staff member may be impaired. By treating the staff member the same as you did prior to the incident, you are showing that it was the act, not the person, that was punished.

Common Mistakes

Mistakes are common in imposing discipline. The nurse may either be apologetic in handing out discipline or may bawl the offender out. The following serve as examples of each:

Apologetic Discipline

NURSE-MANAGER: I hate to seem like a meany, Miss Hanson, but the nursing supervisor expects me to enforce the rules. I'm really sorry that I have to do this.

STAFF MEMBER (*thinking to herself*): Miss Hag thinks the rule is dumb, *or* Miss Hag doesn't have much backbone, *or* Who does she think she's kidding?

Personal Bawling Out

NURSE-MANAGER: I'm getting pretty tired of your slack standards. I've told you repeatedly to keep your IVs on time. What kind of a nurse are you anyway? You certainly aren't the kind of nurse I want working on this unit. You had better start shaping up if you want to keep your job.

In the second example, the discipline is much too personal. There is no need to rub the staff member's nose in dirt. Instead, correct the behavior, assume that the staff member will improve, and write a memo.

Grievance Handling with Union Personnel

In 1974 an amendment to the Taft-Hartley Act made nonprofit health-care facilities subject to the national labor laws. Hospital employees were thus allowed to become unionized.

Generally employees join a union when they feel that they are not being satisfied by the employer. Employees who feel that they are not being treated well by management seek out unionization as a form of power in dealing with management. Because more and more hospital employees are being unionized, the nurse-manager needs knowledge of the ramifications of managing unionized staff members.

Through collective bargaining at the local level the union and hospital administration agree on a contract which specifies wages, hours, work rules, and other conditions of employment. This contract is a legal document about which the nurse-manager needs to be fully informed. In-service education programs or the personnel department should provide nurse-managers with the details of the contract.

It is understood by union and management alike that the signing of a labor contract does not automatically take care of all labor-relations problems that may arise. A grievance procedure, which is part of the contract, provides one means of settling difficulties. The contract states how complaints are to be resolved between union members and the health-care administrators. Most grievances are filed against management.

An example of how a grievance procedure might work is as follows: Mrs. Sherman, an LPN, is upset with the schedule she will be working during the next month. She feels that it is less desirable than the schedules the other LPNs will be working. Her first step in the grievance procedure would be to talk with her manager informally. If this fails she could ask the steward to intercede. The stewards police the labor contract and ensure that managers do not violate its provisions [1]. It is through stewards that formal complaints or grievances are made against management. The steward would attempt to correct the problem by talking with the manager. If this fails, the steward writes a formal complaint to be given to the next level of management, which could be the nursing supervisor. If this also fails, Mrs. Sherman could request that a committee made up of union and management representatives review the grievance. If the results continue to be unfavorable to Mrs. Sherman and if the union officials feel further grievance procedure to be appropriate, the problem is presented to an arbitrator. An arbitrator is a neutral person who hears the case presented by labor and management and resolves the problem by offering a solution which is binding to both.

Agency administrators also need protection against inappropriate actions by unionized subordinates. A portion of the contract is devoted to guidelines on discipline. In the contract there will be a list of inappropriate acts and their associated penalties, and there will be an explanation of due process [6]. The nurse-manager needs to document everything in accordance with procedures in the union contract.

P. King [4] gives seven common laws against which all arbitrators seem to check all discipline cases. They are as follows:

1. Make the rule reasonable.
2. Stay out of private lives.
3. Don't keep rules in your hat.

4. Correct—don't punish.
5. Make the punishment uniform.
6. Don't double up on punishment.
7. Grant the benefit of the doubt.

The grievance procedure is a valuable protection for the employee. The nurse-manager needs to read and fully understand any union/management contract so that the rights of union members are protected and the hospital is not subject to lengthy and costly labor disputes.

Common Disciplinary Problems

Let us look at some of the more common disciplinary problems that we find in nursing situations:

1. *The Absentee:* You have probably had staff members who are chronically absent from work. Equally aggravating are the staff members who neither come to work nor call to say they will not be at work. Weekends especially can be notorious for absenteeism of staff members. What can be done about this problem? A procedure should exist, be known to employees, and be enforced that spells out: (1) when to call, (2) whom to call, and (3) what happens when there is no call. A policy needs to be written as to how many days of absenteeism is unreasonable. The chronic absentee who is away from work unreasonably should be discharged. Warning the employee of probable discharge should precede the discharge.
2. *The Loafer:* Staff members who are present at work but are not doing their job are another common problem. Night nurses may even work with staff members who sleep on the job. Here, again, a policy should exist and be enforced. The wrongdoer must be corrected and warned. The manager can keep a record of the offenses to back up the cause for any additional discipline.
3. *The Staff Member Working Under Par:* A job description must exist for each category of employee. If a staff member does not work up to the standards spelled out in the job description, and training and constructive criticism have failed, then the nurse-manager must show where poor performance exists. Once again written memos of examples of behavior are helpful in substantiating your charge against the staff member.

4. *The Rebel:* Occasionally we encounter staff members who refuse an aspect of their assignment. For example, an aide may refuse to admit a patient or take care of a particular patient. Find out the reason for the refusal. If the reason does not "hold water," then disciplinary measures are needed following the principles stated earlier.

Conclusions

Basically, discipline is a form of training. Failure to keep staff members informed may be the cause of the disciplinary problem. It takes more than one-way communication, however. Staff members need to regard the rules as acceptable. Managers must initiate discipline by winning acceptance of the standards.

For discipline to be accepted, the rules must be known to all the staff members, and penalties for disregarding rules must be consistent. Discipline helps staff members recognize their job requirements and if done impersonally can build a stronger group that renders better patient care.

Group Session

1. What occurs when the nurse-manager is inconsistent in handling disciplinary situations?
2. What happens when two head nurses on two different units handle similar disciplinary problems in completely different ways?
3. Why have you failed as a manager and leader if you do not maintain discipline on your unit?
4. Do a relatively few individuals cause most of the disciplinary problems in your school or agency? Why? What characteristics do they have in common?
5. What happens when the nurse-manager overlooks that Miss Jones, NA, stays away from work three days without calling in to inform the manager?
   a. What effect does this have on Miss Jones?
   b. What effect does it have on the other staff members?
   c. How does this decrease the nurse-manager's effectiveness?
6. Suppose an RN has been making frequent small mistakes. Is it better for the manager to: (1) discuss each mistake separately as it occurs, or (2) discuss the RN's overall performance with her from time to time?
7. What are the established "rules of conduct" in your school or agency? Who formulated them? Do the managers or instructors know what they are? Do all the staff members or students know what they are?
   a. How do they know?

b. What steps have been taken to ensure that they understand the policies?
c. Are they enforced? If not, why not?
8. Does your school or agency have an established disciplinary policy? Does a procedure exist for implementing it?
9. What are the criteria for dismissing an employee or student in your agency or school?
a. Do you know?
b. Do the employees or students know?
c. Is there a chance for appeal? To whom is the appeal made?

References

1. Alexander, K. G.   Union structure and bargaining structure. *Labor Law J.* 24:164, 1973.
2. Argyris, C.   *Executive Leadership*. New York: Harper & Row, 1953. P. xiii.
3. Cassels, L.   Discipline: Key to high morale. *Nation's Business* 47:82–91, Nov. 1959.
4. King, P.   Tips to successful discipline. *Factory Management and Maintenance* 116:78–87, June 1958.
5. Strauss, G., and Sayles, L.   *Personnel: The Human Problems of Management* (3rd ed.). Englewood Cliffs, N.J.: Prentice-Hall, 1972. Pp. 264–282.
6. Werther, W. B., Jr., and Lockhart, C. A.   *Labor Relations in the Health Professions*. Boston: Little, Brown, 1976.

Suggested Reading

Anderson, M., and Farran, C.   We are accountable. (#16-1626) New York: National League for Nursing, 1976. Pp. 147–168.
Bennett, R. and MacRobert, R.   Building skills in discipline and grievance handling. Part 1—*Hosp. Top.* 53:8, Jan./Feb. 1975. Part 2—*Hosp. Top.* 53:50, March/April 1975.
Bryant, Y.   Labor relations in health care institutions: An analysis of Public Law 93-360. *J. Nurs. Adm.* 8:28, March 1978.
Davis, K.   Steps toward a more flexible disciplinary policy. *Personnel* 38:52–56, May/June 1961.
Hamil, E. M.   Conflict management . . . flight, fight, negotiate. (#52-1677) New York: National League for Nursing, 1977. Pp. 1–6.
Herron, I., Nash, P., Roberts, L., Lewis, L., and Bishop, A.   Labor-management issues in the health care fields. (#21-1624) New York: National League for Nursing, 1976. Pp. 1–59.
Knutson, K. E., and Robertson, P.   The disciplinary conference letter. *Superv. Nurse* 7:10, March 1976.
Marriner, A.   Discipline of personnel. *Superv. Nurse* 7:15, Nov. 1976.
Petersen, D. J., and Halstead, E. G.   The arbitration of cases involving improper professional conduct in the health care industry. *A.A.N.A. J.* 45:189, April 1977.

12. Communication

Communication is the integration process of management. Every chapter in this book deals with theories and techniques of management, and you will find that they all involve relating to other people. In this chapter some of the basic communication tools important to effective management are isolated and their application to working relationships is explored.

Communication Skills

A manager fills many roles. Among them are ambassador, consultant, innovator, boss, disciplinarian, and practitioner. All these roles require communication skills. Managerial communications encompass all types of communicating. The manager must listen, read, write memos and notes, fill out forms and requisitions, and talk to others. The manager is actually in a pivotal position in an organization and must articulate not only the purposes of the organization to the staff but also the needs and problems of the staff to the organization's administrative personnel. Let us examine some of the communication skills inherent in the manager's many roles.

An ambassador must be able to listen, to know what to say and when to communicate. This knowledge stems from understanding people and events so that communication will be effective for each situation. Nurse-ambassadors have to know how to phrase their communication so that patients and staff members will understand what they are saying. Managers have to know how to interpret what is being said to them so that their responses will be appropriate. Tact and diplomacy are criteria for communicating to personnel from other departments, patients, families, and staff members. These characteristics enable the nurse-managers to develop common understanding and cooperative relationships among all those with whom they work.

Innovators often have ideas that are new and different. Therefore, managers who are also innovators must be able to channel the thinking of others along their line of reasoning. This requires that innovators develop acceptance of innovative ideas by being persuasive, logical, and patient. Communication must reflect these characteristics. In nursing, it is sometimes difficult to gain the nursing staff's acceptance of new ways of doing things, because the tried and true method seems to work well. Innovators in this situation must lead people to understand the purposes for change and to become involved in the growth process. Communication is very important in this process.

To be boss and to be disciplinarian require that managers be able to express themselves with sincerity and directness. The communications required of a boss and of a disciplinarian are related. The boss must be able to give clear, meaningful directions. The nurse-manager, for example, must succinctly outline the care a nurse's aide is to give a patient so that the aide understands what has to be done. The disciplinarian must be able to cite definite and pertinent events that define an individual's personal responsibility for doing or not doing what should have been accomplished. The nurse's aide, for example, must be told why the manager is not satisfied with the patient care given through the use of specific examples if the communication is to be meaningful. Both the boss and the disciplinarian roles require that the manager assess events and performance of workers through listening as well as observing. Both roles require a constructive approach in communication so that improved performance will result. Both require that the manager be open in communication so that the workers feel that even though their performance requires improvement, they are supported and understood by the manager.

Use of terminology in nursing is important in fostering common understanding in the specialized field of health care. The professional nurse must be able to articulate needs and goals of patient care to other professionals in the hospital and community in a way that fosters acceptance, respect, and cooperation. A common language among the health-related professionals is the basis for common understanding and cooperation. In addition, nurse-managers must be concerned with proper use of terminology peculiar to the particular organization in which they work. The managers must be able to use and interpret standard forms, requisitions, and memos for communicating with other departments. It is important to understand and recognize the nuances of communication peculiar to the organization—the unwritten policies and the accepted routes for communicating used within an organization which have their basis in the way people work together rather than in formal policy. All these organizational communications serve to integrate the work of employees in an organization.

Communication Networks

In an organization networks of communication are delineated by the general organizational structure. The networks are established to channel the continuous flow of information. This flow is contiguous with coordination of efforts and cooperation. Generally, the networks are formed on the basis of who needs what information. People in the organization relate to the networks in two major ways—they impart information and they receive information.

Numerous methods can be used to transmit information in an organization. When the information can be consistently categorized, a stable format can be devised to provide a means for "automatic" communication. The format may be a report form, a checklist, or any procedure that outlines necessary information. The networks are used to channel this information according to which persons need it and when they require it for their work.

Information that cannot be categorized, such as that concerned with solving problems, planning, and developing new ideas, takes place through personal contacts, conferences, and through written memos. In this instance the networks of communication serve to define which persons should be involved in these activities.

The major networks (which are often overlapping) with which the nurse-manager is involved in a health-care agency usually include the following:

Nurse-patient
Nurse-staff member
Nurse-supervisor
Nurse-other hospital employees
Nurse-doctor
Nurse-family and agencies in the community

All communication that takes place through these networks is concerned with the work of the organization and with the workers' needs to communicate. Managers in various positions determine how these networks can be used, what methods best suit transmission of specific information, and what they will do with the information they receive. A major management responsibility then is making sure that communication flows along the networks and that the information received is made useful.

Communication is important to workers in an organization. Those who impart information should consider that what is heard, understood, and believed by other persons is determined to a large extent by the receivers' systems of thought. The person who imparts information realizes that if the information is necessary for work, it must also be valid and pertinent to that work and should be obtained by the receiver at an appropriate time. By the same token, those who receive information must make an effort to understand and interpret what has been communicated.

Nurse-Patient Communication

Let us consider some of the techniques of communication that are appropriate to specific communication networks in the nurse's realm of management. In your study of nursing you have discovered that patient care requires sensitivity to patient needs and thoughtful planning to meet the needs assessed by the nurse. Among the techniques used by nurses to accomplish this are interviewing, reading, discussing patient care with others, conferring with the doctors, the patients, and the patients' families, and imparting information through explanations of pamphlets, brochures, films, slide-tape presentations, and other illustrations or diagrams that can be used for teaching patients.

Through your study of nursing you have also learned that many factors are involved in any given communication. You learned, for example, that communication takes place through the written word, verbally, and through nonverbal communications such as bodily position, facial expression, and gestures. You gradually gained skill in looking beneath the surface of any communication for meanings and implications because you increasingly became aware of the fact that superficial communication is sometimes misleading. True therapeutic communication is concerned with "crawling into another's skin," reaching the depths of the other person's reactions, and supporting that person in adjustment and adaptation.

Just as nurse-patient communications must have depth to be effective, so do nurse-staff communications. Social amenities are not sufficient for interaction among a manager and staff members when they are working toward progress and goal achievement. They are also not sufficient for developing innovative methods for giving health care or for facilitating growth of staff members. Therefore, nurse-managers should apply all the knowledge and skill they have gained in nurse-patient communications to their communications with staff members.

Nurse-Staff Communication

Leaders have great power to shape how others interpret information they receive and how they analyze events that occur. The major way leaders influence others is by their own "transmissions." Leaders of groups bear the responsibility for integrating all communication pertinent to the group so that it is indeed useful to the work. They place this integrated information in context for group members; the way the leaders communicate, the attitudes demonstrated, the way information is organized, and the methods used to present information all affect how the communication will be received by the staff members. Staff members' interpretation is colored also by the way they perceive that leaders want them to react to their communication.

SENSITIVITY TO STAFF

Attitudes are extremely important in shaping the morale of staff members. Cooperation is enhanced if the leader of the group remembers some nonacademic but basic facts. First of all, no individuals like to hear negative things about themselves: Do you? How do you react when someone tells you that Mrs. X thinks that you don't listen, are not efficient, or that you are lazy? Another fact is that all people want their efforts and abilities to be appreciated—feedback is needed to support one's self-concept. Although staff members may believe that they are doing a good job, they need to know for sure. When those in authority or those whose opinions staff members value also think they are doing a good job, then they are supported in self-knowledge. For example, in preceding chapters it has been stated that people, when allowed to participate in decision-making, are more likely to be committed to carrying out the decisions because they accept and understand them. Basically, the manager who allows others to participate in decision-making and who then uses their decisions is recognizing staff members' worth, intelligence, and capabilities.

The third point to remember is that everybody wants to be "in the right." Making errors is considered inappropriate behavior that can exclude an individual from a group. The manager who communicates effectively reduces the probability of errors' being made because of misunderstandings about what is expected or through misinterpretations about what has been said.

Personality conflicts among staff members occur—in fact, some think that they are inevitable. The manager must realize that when they do occur, conflict can be localized to those most directly involved. The manager can support the staff in working through conflicts and can act as a mediator in conflicts by being positive about each person and by demonstrating respect for them and for their work. However, the manager must remember that each person has the most intimate understanding of his or her own feelings and problems and must accept and work through relationships in a personal way.

ASSESSING COMMUNICATION NEEDS
Managers have to be sensitive to the staff members and must assess their needs for communication. The network of manager-staff relationships relates to the work as well as to the staff's personal needs for communication. Managers should examine the total scope of information that the staff members need to do their jobs and then should devise definite methods or formats suitable to impart this information. In addition, nurse-managers have to consider what kind of information they need from the staff and then must similarly devise methods to obtain this through the communication networks.

Beginning managers are sometimes reluctant to tap this network's potential because of basic uncertainties about their ability to fill the managerial role. A study conducted in Pillsbury installations [1] demonstrated the importance of the leader's communication and revealed that good communications contribute to favorable employee attitudes. Employees indicated that good communication involved providing them with the information they wanted, quickly and through channels they preferred. The majority of employees preferred to get information from their own supervisors. We can apply the findings of this study to nursing management. How do you relate to the staff members? Do you provide information to them when they need it? Do you communicate enough?

If the manager of a group does not provide members of the group with adequate information, they will find their own. This means that group members will be susceptible to rumors about their work and about their status. If they do not know "how it actually is," they will decide for themselves which of the rumors are true. Similarly, if rumors are not available, the staff members will posit "how it is." They will consider what they think is happening according to the information they have. The result is often a misconstruing of information to far more negative conclusions than even the most punitive of managers could entertain. People tend to be hard on themselves when they are speculating about matters that affect them personally, and they often conjure up unrealistic problems and feelings through their speculation. Because of this, the manager who finally does communicate information will have to work through all the rumors and speculation before the staff members will understand and accept what is being said to them.

Communication with Individual Staff Members

Managers must talk to their staff members regularly and must make each communication meaningful in order to achieve a continuous development of common understanding and interpretation between themselves and the staff members. As the common understanding grows, the communication becomes more effective, and eventually the manager can more easily and correctly discern what is on the employee's mind while the employee can just as easily determine what is on the manager's mind. Have you ever experienced this type of common understanding with members of your family or with friends?

Much has been written in previous chapters about how to delegate work, how to give directions, and how to evaluate the performance of others. All these activities can be considered one-to-one relationships between the managers and the staff members. Managers should remember that in conducting all these activities they must talk to the other persons, not around or through them. Have you ever received direction from a group leader through someone else rather than from that manager? Or have you ever talked to some other people, all the while thinking that they were uninterested in what you were saying—and perhaps did not even hear you? A building relationship between manager and staff member can be maintained by referring to previous communication and achievement and by leading up to the next step in every interaction.

A BUILDING RELATIONSHIP

Such a building relationship is illustrated by the story of Jane Abel, a new nurse's aide. The group leader, Carol Inlow, had a short conference with Jane when she first came to work. In this conference she asked her what she expected from her job, what she wanted to accomplish, and how she could help her the most. At first Jane was reluctant to answer, saying that she did not yet know enough about the work. Eventually, Carol found that Jane was particularly uncomfortable about what to say to patients and about how the other staff members would treat her. Carol planned for Jane to spend the first week of orientation to the unit with a nurse who was particularly adept at communication skills and who understood Jane's needs to be oriented to the group and to patient care on that unit.

Each time that Carol gave Jane her assignment, she would be particularly careful to tell her human-interest anecdotes about her patients. When Jane reported to her, she would ask her to relate her feelings about the patients and to describe what she had learned by working with the experienced nurse. Carol made a point of discussing patients' reactions with her and also supported the positive things she had accomplished by complimenting her, both alone and in group meetings. As a result, Jane felt that she could talk to Carol, that she was learning how to communicate better, and that when she questioned her own interaction, Carol would help her determine what she should have said or done, without indicating that she should have known better in the first place. In this instance the group leader created a situation in which she and the staff member were free to communicate about a personal problem, because the climate had been set for learning.

WRITTEN RECORDS OF COMMUNICATION

The manager should keep a written record of interaction with staff members. For example, Carol kept notes on Jane's daily progress in improving her communication skills. From the last month's notes she found that Jane was less fearful of other staff members, noting that she increasingly had asked for help, initiated group activities on three recent occasions, and offered to help others consistently during the previous week. Carol's notes also indicated that Jane communicated more easily with people who were older or younger than she, but that she had the most difficulty with those in her own peer group. Carol might have been able to "feel" that these things were so by remembering what Jane did. However, with good notes she could point to specific incidents that objectively supported her feelings.

Communication with Staff as a Group
THE STAFF CONFERENCE

Perhaps the most common technique used by managers to work with staff members collectively is the staff meeting or the conference. When staff members are assembled for a conference, the manager has to make sure that they know why the conference is being held, that they feel comfortable in participating in the conference, and that the conference is useful to them in their work. A conference usually progresses through phases of climate setting, of orientation, of participants' expectations for the conference, information sharing or collecting, group participation in planning priorities for action, and determination of how to follow up on what has been discussed or decided.

GUIDELINES FOR CONDUCTING CONFERENCES
The conference or meeting is one of the best opportunities for a manager to ascertain what staff members are thinking about and how they are relating to one another. Some pointers about conducting successful conferences follow:

1. Inform staff members about the purpose of the conference in advance so that they will be prepared.
2. Set a definite time for the conference as well as a time limit, and make sure that the conference starts and ends on time.
3. Be prepared for the conference. If you are holding a conference to impart information, think through your approach to the topic, your presentation of the information, and your conclusions about how the information should be used. Do not expect the staff to apply the information, especially if it is new, after just hearing a presentation of facts. You must explain how they should apply the information if you want them do draw the same conclusions that you have drawn.
4. Arrange materials for demonstration or for illustration in advance and make sure that any equipment you are using is in working order. Graphics are helpful in presenting complicated information, and an explanation of new equipment is more meaningful if people can actually see how it works.
5. If you are having a conference for the purpose of problem-solving by the staff, you must be prepared to speak on the topic as a consultant for the group. This requires just as much preparation as actual presentation of material does, if not more.
6. Solicit participation from group members. Ask them what they think about the topic, listen to what they say, and use the information they put forth in your comments.
7. Each conference should be summarized at the end. The summary should include comments made by participants to demon-

strate the value of their contributions, as well as a summary of what has been accomplished during the conference.

8. If the conference is one of a series conducted for the purpose of developing plans or special projects, begin each session with a review of what happened previously. At the end of the conference the summary should indicate what is to happen next in order to establish goals for the next session.

9. Plan the meetings or conferences to meet definite needs of the staff for doing work better. If the topics are relevant to the workers, they will contribute more effectively to the conferences. Refer to discussions, solutions to problems, or plans that have been made in the conference when it is appropriate in performing daily work activities. This helps staff members appreciate the importance of the conferences and makes them part of the work rather than extracurricular activities.

10. If conferences are being held to develop a project or plan, provide staff members with an assignment so that they can contribute to the sessions in a positive way. Merely talking about a topic for problem-solving soon exhausts the staff's ideas. They must bring new input to the conferences if they are to be "growth" sessions.

11. When assignments have been given for conferences, allow sufficient time for staff members to complete the assignment before the conference is held. Sessions should be close enough together to provide motivation for doing the assignment while it is fresh. Otherwise staff members tend to rationalize about doing the "homework" because there is plenty of time and it can always be done later.

12. Keep minutes or notes about each meeting or conference. In this way you can remember what has taken place and staff members can refer to notes if there are questions about decisions that have been made by the group. Keeping good notes prevents staff from belaboring the same points over and over again; minutes also help staff members maintain consistency in applying what has been learned in the conferences. A written record of meetings and conferences is also helpful to demonstrate progress, or lack of progress, toward accomplishing the goals of the sessions. Managers have many interruptions in their train of thought during the course of one day and deal with a myriad of different problems over a span of time. Notes help the manager remember what has happened; by reviewing notes objectively, the manager can determine patterns in behavior and

in events. This review serves as an evaluative measure to provide input on which future decisions can be based.

COMMITTEES

Many of the concepts that apply to conducting and to participating in conferences also apply to committees. Committees are used for decision-making, to gain employee acceptance of new ideas, and to promote communication among employees, or to establish or maintain relationships with consumers or community agency representatives. You may be a member of a committee comprising nurses, or you may be appointed to a committee comprising many different types of health professionals. In some instances you may be the only nurse on the committee. Organizations typically have many different kinds of committees; some may be temporary (ad hoc) and others may be standing committees with changing or rotating appointment of members. The standing committees are often a part of the organizational structure and may have operational responsibilities.

Committees serve to coordinate efforts in an organization and to elicit cooperation among employees through participation in committee decision-making. Productive and active committees can be a mechanism for challenging employees and for stimulating motivation. Committees are groups, and their effectiveness is therefore determined to some extent by the expertise of the members, by the members' ability to use group process to work constructively together, and by the usefulness and applicability of the committee's activities to the organization's work.

Members of committees are often selected from among employees for a purpose. You may be selected for a specific committee because that committee needs a nurse-representative. As a member of a committee you often represent a group of employees—a group of nurses or the group that composes the staff of your unit. Initially you may feel uncomfortable if you are appointed to a committee made up of people you do not know or of employees who represent administration or other professional groups such as doctors. It is important for you to realize that you have an important role as a member of the committee and that your contribution to committee activities is of value. In addition, your particular nursing expertise on committees with "mixed membership" ensures that the nursing point of view is considered in committee decisions.

To participate effectively in such committees, it is necessary that you do your "homework" and that you know the issues involved and how those issues impact on nursing. It is prudent for a committee member to discover how others in the organization feel about the committee's activities and to learn from others how to deal with interaction among committee members. Participation in active committees can be a valuable learning experience that serves to broaden your perspective by sharing ideas and concepts with others. Through committee membership, you will find that you meet people you would not have known otherwise. You can learn from these people, just as they can learn from you.

Written Communication

All the other networks of communication in the nurse-manager's realm are similar to the nurse-patient and nurse-staff interactions. The major differences are that the farther the network is removed from the immediate nursing-care unit, the more predesigned formats for conveying information are used. An example of a format is a referral form that the nurses might use for the Visiting Nurse Association. This form includes basic questions that are important for continuity of care. The necessary information can be written in a uniform manner. Usually it includes information that is common to all patients; this can be presented in the form of a checklist. Other portions of the form require information specific to the given patient. These forms supplement oral communication and can be retained for the patient's record for future reference.

EFFECTIVENESS OF YOUR WRITTEN COMMUNICATION

When completing referral forms, or in preparing written communication, there are some simple questions that you can use to evaluate the effectiveness of your communication. First, is it readable? Is it thoughtful? Have you included the most important facts about the patient? If you were reading these comments without previous knowledge of the patient, could you form a clear picture of the patient's needs? Are your comments appropriate for the situation? Are they objective? Are they realistic? Is the information you have given correct? Can specific information be checked if necessary? Could you have written your comments in fewer words while still retaining the meaning?

VALUE OF WRITTEN COMMUNICATIONS

Writing memos, explanations, or narrative statements requires the art of conciseness and clarity. All the previous questions are applicable to anything that the manager writes for other people's use. It is important to note that everything committed to writing forms a record that can be retained. The record can serve as a check to see if work has been accomplished, as a means for evaluating whether something should or should not be done, or as a source of ideas that state your problems or position about a given topic. Writing is a valuable tool in an organization because of the great number of demands upon people's time and energy. Although it is sometimes easier to call and discuss a problem with someone on the phone, the written memo serves as a reminder that could jog memories. There seems to be a natural tendency for people to respect the written word, so that if you wish to make a greater impression you are more likely to do so in writing.

THE REPORT

A common means of communication in organizations is the report. This may be written or verbal. Many reports are verbal and can be recorded for information retrieval. Staff members report to their managers, the managers report to their managers, and so on along the scalar chain.

A good report includes an introduction to the topic, succinct discussion of events and related problems, and presentation of facts in logical sequence. Uniformity of order when giving a report helps the listener clarify what is being said. The report should be given clearly without distortion. This means that the speaker's voice should be audible and that extraneous information should be deleted. The latter is important to prevent information overload for the listeners.

Two major types of information are important in reporting: (1) information gleaned from observations and (2) information that can be documented. The person reporting should differentiate between the two so that the listener knows which information is subject to differences in perception and which information is fixed and definite. Again, reports are developed to give the listener the information needed to accomplish work and to provide for continuity.

REVIEW OF FORMATS OF WRITTEN COMMUNICATION

Formats used to facilitate communication should be reviewed periodically to ensure that they continue to fulfill their functions. Everyone involved in use of the format should be included in the evaluation review to make sure that all opinions about the effectiveness of the communication for all persons along the network are considered. Subtle changes are continually taking place in organizations because new employees use different methods and have different styles; therefore, ideas that were in vogue yesterday may not be stylish today, and new methods may have been initiated because of external factors such as legislative requirements for some organizational activity. These are a few of the reasons why periodic review is necessary.

DEVELOPING EFFECTIVE PERSONAL COMMUNICATION
When nurses are involved in changing the health-care system, either through development of their particular role in an organization or through group interaction with persons from related disciplines, they must learn to identify and to articulate their thoughts in a sophisticated way. This means that nurses must first of all be well informed about current events in nursing and related health-care activities. They must be cognizant of the issues inherent in the planning, and they must draw independent conclusions about the meaning of all this information. Nurses should go through the process of information analysis before attending meetings so that their contribution to the meeting will be meaningful.

One of the best ways to clarify thoughts is to participate in discussions. Sometimes merely saying something out loud helps one realize what it means. Have you ever changed your mind or clarified a thought in midsentence? For some people writing out ideas is even better than talking. Try writing out your thoughts concerning a specific activity you deal with in patient care. Write down the purpose of the activity, the methods used to accomplish the purpose, and the results of the activity. Place what you have written in a secure place and let it cool. Then go back a week later and read it. How does it sound to you one week later? How would you change what you have written? This process is helpful not only in thinking through an idea but also in forming a sense of objectivity.

A good question for the nurse-manager is How can you explain the results of your staff members' work? Try telling someone what you have achieved during the past month. Can you remember events you were most proud of? Or those that bothered you the most? Are certain events clouded in your mind? A written diary of your evaluation of the results of each day's activities is of considerable help in defining results over a period of time. From it you can identify a pattern of good and bad performance. As you read, question: Is there uniformity in the way people behave at work and in the way you manage? Can you identify consistency in successes or problems? Are the activities you have described appropriate to the needs of the situation? Could you have avoided some difficulties with better planning? How could you improve?

Effective communication incorporates a sense of curiosity with a sense of propriety. Managers will acquire information if their minds are open and questioning. Managers should keep in mind a saying the author once read: "Keep your mind open, something might fall into it." The sense of propriety serves to ensure that the communication networks are used to best advantage in the most appropriate manner. Essentially, this is part of the ability to get along with others. If you, as manager, respect others' needs for information, they will in turn respect your own needs.

Conclusions

Communication is essential to stability in the organization. Staff members do not like to feel that they are in a vacuum; they need to know that they will be listened to and that they will receive information. Effective communication helps workers feel confident in their working relationships. This in turn helps workers feel secure about themselves and about their work. When people are confident and secure, they can better meet the challenges for progressively improving their abilities to do their jobs.

Study Questions

1. In a group of students identify all the techniques and tools that are used in the nurse-manager's network of communication. Examine all of these tools to determine:
   a. Their purpose
   b. Their value for communicating
   c. Results of their use
2. Outline a series of topics for meetings that you wish to conduct with your staff for the purpose of:
   a. Imparting information
   b. Sharing information
   c. Improving patient care
3. Keep a diary of all your communications as a manager for a period of one week. Classify these according to communication:
   a. About direct patient care
   b. About staff members' needs and problems
   c. With the administrative staff

  d. With the doctors
  e. With other departments
  f. With patients and their families
  g. With other agencies
  Within each classification determine if the communication was effective, if it took unncessary time, and if it could be better organized. Evaluate whether the communication you imparted and that you received was adequate.
4. Isolate one patient and draw the networks of communication you were involved with in caring for the patient, placing yourself in the middle of the communication networks. Include communication that you initiated and communication you received.
5. Evaluate how communication networks in an organization might be illustrated in:
  a. A bureaucratic organizational structure
  b. A decentralized organizational structure
  c. A matrix organization

Reference

1. Gefland, L.   Communicate through your supervisors. *Harvard Bus. Rev.* 48:101–104, Nov./Dec. 1970.

Suggested Reading

American Nurses Association Clinical Conference, 1969, Minneapolis/ Atlanta.   New York: Appleton-Century-Crofts, 1970.
Coffin, R. A.   *The Communicator.* New York: American Management Association, 1975.
Egan, G.   *Interpersonal Living.* Monterey, Cal.: Brooks/Cole, 1975.
Egan, G.   *The Skilled Helper.* Monterey, Cal.: Brooks/Cole, 1976.
Hemalt, M.D., and Mackert, M. E.   Factual medical records protect hospitals, practitioners, patients. *Hospitals* 51:13, July 1, 1977.
Kron, T.   *Communication in Nursing* (2nd ed.). Philadelphia: Saunders, 1972.
Matson, F. W., and Montagu, A. (Eds.)   *The Human Dialogue: Perspectives on Communication.* New York: The Free Press, 1967.
Price, E. M.   *Learning Needs of Registered Nurses.* New York: Teachers College Press, Columbia University, 1967.
Redman, B.   *The Process of Patient Teaching in Nursing* (3rd ed.). St. Louis: Mosby, 1976.
Ujhely, G.   *Determinants of the Nurse-Patient Relationship.* New York: Springer, 1968.
Wiley, L.   Communications: Understanding the gravity of the situation. *Nursing '76* 6:4, April 1976.

III. Case Studies

This section contains cases that are designed to give you practice in managerial thinking. Management is complex and requires synthesis of many different theories and principles as they apply to a given situation. In working through these cases you can develop a perspective of the manager's role in analyzing situations. You can define priorities, develop plans for action, and make decisions that are based on the theories and principles presented in the first two parts of this book. These cases can provide you with a model for defining and analyzing the situations encountered in the work situation. Management of patient care in an organization involves working through many similar "cases" that are full of challenges and problems to solve. Your experiences in management can be considered cases that require thoughtful decision-making and that allow you to reflect on the impact that you can make through application of management theories and principles.

The case studies presented in this section have been designed to provide you with situations you might encounter in the work situation. Each of the case studies included has been developed to emphasize one component of management theory, but, as with real-life situations, their solution is not limited to a discrete aspect of management. Instead you must synthesize the theories and principles of management in solving these cases. As with most management situations there are no right or wrong solutions. Solving the cases depends on developing a rationale for action based on determination of the dynamics that are taking place in each situation. You can become familiar with managerial roles in solving these cases.

Practice in management gives you an opportunity to develop a perspective of a manager's role and behaviors. One of the most difficult adjustments you may make as a newly graduated nurse in a first job is in becoming a manager in the context of an organization. Your previous experiences in management may have been limited to direct patient care. Even though you may have completed patient-care experiences in a variety of health-care agencies, you may not have belonged to the organization as an employee. In your first position you become part of the organization and must learn to function within that organization in a managerial role. These cases, and others that you may develop from your own experiences, will help you to develop the broadened perspective necessary for assuming your new managerial role.

Amerton Hospital Case

Amerton General Hospital is a 350-bed hospital located in the city of Amerton, which has a population of 95,000. The majority of patients served at Amerton General are self-supporting and have hospitalization insurance. About five percent of the in-patients are on welfare. The salaries of the majority of hospital personnel are slightly below the average income within the community. Both professional and other employees of the hospital are largely recruited from Amerton and the nearby towns. Amerton General is the larger of two hospitals in the area.

Four North, which is one of the 11 units at Amerton General, has 36 patient beds and comprises four private rooms, eight semiprivate rooms, and four wards of four beds each. It is primarily a general thoracic surgery unit. The average length of stay for a patient is 12 days. Usually one preoperative day is used for tests, one day for operation, and the remaining days for intensive postoperative care and convalescing care.

Mrs. Webster, Head Nurse

The unit's leader is Mrs. Webster, aged 47, who is the head nurse. She has held this position for five years. She had worked 10 years as a staff nurse prior to and between the births of her three children. Mrs. Webster takes pride in being neat and precise. She enjoys her position of authority and relates easily to physicians and those of equal and superior positions in the hospital hierarchy. She sees her role as that of a manager and devotes the majority of her time to making out time schedules, keeping supply rooms stocked and orderly, attending meetings, and promoting smooth functioning between 4N and other hospital units and departments.

On occasional holidays and weekends, when only one other registered nurse is working on the unit, Mrs. Webster functions as team leader for 18 patients. As a team leader, she passes medications to patients and delegates all other aspects of patient care to team members. She does very little follow-up to see that assignments are completed, but when she reports to the next shift, she almost always knows what tests have been completed and what changes have been made in the patients' treatments. During the week, when Mrs. Webster makes "rounds" on the patients, they are primarily social in nature. At times patients express problems to her, some of which she occasionally follows through to solve.

Mrs. Webster believes in team nursing and is especially interested in team conferences. Occasionally she enjoys presenting nursing or medical knowledge to the team at a conference. For example, Mrs. Webster often conducts conferences for teaching team members about a subject, such as cancer of the larynx.

Mrs. Webster is known to others as being somewhat egotistical, but she is well liked as a person. Her actual expertise at nursing is difficult to evaluate as she rarely becomes involved in direct patient care.

Patients are generally pleased with the care they receive on 4N. Mrs. Webster is well known in the community, and people associate her self-confidence with a well-run patient-care unit. In contrast, some of the other units in Amerton General have reputations for being disorganized or sloppy.

Staff Members

On a typical day on 4N the following events transpire. At 7:00 A.M. the night nurse gives a report to the day shift. There is a total of 36 patients on the unit today. Mrs. Webster has divided the staff into two teams:

Team 1	*Team 2*
Team Leader: Mrs. Kent, RN	Team Leader: Mrs. Crawford
Miss Winter, RN	Mrs. Evans, LPN
Mrs. Cooper, aide	Mrs. Green, LPN
Mrs. Taber, aide	Miss Allen, aide

TEAM 1: PERSONNEL

Mrs. Kent is very pleasant to work with. Her nursing care is good but could be more complete. She enjoys chatting with the team members and visitors and allows herself to be away from the patients for 30 to 45 minutes at a time while she chats socially. Mrs. Kent is four months pregnant.

Miss Winter was graduated from nursing school two years ago and has worked on 4N since graduation. She enjoys nursing and gives thorough nursing care. She prefers caring for a group of patients rather than being a team leader. Mrs. Cooper, nurse's aide, is energetic and pleasant, but her nursing knowledge is limited. Her observations of patients are incomplete, and she lacks common sense and judgment. She generally asks questions when she does not understand. Mrs. Taber seems lazy and gets by with doing as little work as possible. She is a mother of six and needs to work to help support her family.

TYPICAL DAY: TEAM 1

Mrs. Kent, team leader, begins her day by checking medication cards, pouring and preparing medications, and passing medications to patients. She sees her first patient at 8:30 A.M. She chats briefly with patients as she gives them their medications. Both Mrs. Cooper and Mrs. Taber have taken patients' temperatures and have started giving patients their morning baths and getting them ready for breakfast. Miss Winter, RN, is giving care to an unconscious patient.

After passing medications, Mrs. Kent stops to make herself a snack of crackers and peanut butter. She sits on a stool in the medicine room and chats with anyone who comes in. By 10:30 A.M. Mrs. Cooper and Mrs. Taber have completed the morning care for their patients. Miss Winter is still giving patient care. The patients on Team 1 have received essential physical care only. There has been no patient teaching, patients who need help in ambulation are still in bed, and treatments that are to be done two times on the day shift have not been done once. Blood pressures have been taken.

At 10:30 A.M. Mrs. Kent makes rounds on her team, using Kardex as a guide. She notes that one patient's IV is 100 cc behind schedule and that another patient's Foley catheter is leaking. Three patients ask her for the bedpan as she is making rounds. The aides are nowhere in sight. Mrs. Kent gives the patients the needed care. She makes a list of things that need to be done for the patients and goes to find the team members. Miss Winter is talking with a physician. Mrs. Cooper and Mrs. Taber are taking a coffee break in the conference room. Mrs. Kent asks Mrs. Cooper to do a few things when she finishes her break. Mrs. Cooper agrees pleasantly. When Mrs. Taber is asked to do a few things for patients, she replies, "I'm going to soak Mr. Black's foot just once today. He is such a baby about having the dressing removed. Mrs. Smith won't cough and deep breathe for me. I told her she'd get pneumonia if she didn't. I'll get to that other stuff later." Mrs. Kent does not pursue the issue.

The afternoon finds the team members accomplishing the patient treatments once, ambulating the patients one time each, and doing their charting. It has been a typical day. No one has been rushed to complete her work. The patients seem content and none have complained about their care.

TEAM 2: PERSONNEL

Mrs. Crawford was graduated four years ago from a university nursing program. She worked three years at a medical center hospital in a different state before coming to Amerton. She expects perfection of herself and the team members in meeting patient-care needs. Mrs. Crawford often finds herself upset with the slack standards she observes in team members. She feels that much more could be done to improve the quality of care the patients on 4N are receiving.

Mrs. Evans, LPN, works hard most of the time. She is not consistent, however. She may do an excellent job one day and a poor job the next day. She is moody and calls in sick about twice a month. Mrs. Green, LPN, is somewhat nervous and shows her irritability openly. She can do an excellent job or can loaf and accomplish little. She relates to Miss Winter particularly well and likes to be on the same team with Miss Winter. Miss Allen, nurse's aide, does what she is told in her assignment but never goes beyond those instructions. She resents having any tasks added to her original assignment. She frequently grumbles that her assignment is too heavy but is often observed taking extended coffee and lunch breaks.

TYPICAL DAY: TEAM 2

Mrs. Crawford takes extensive notes during report. Her assignment conference to team members is thorough and complete. Mrs. Evans, LPN, takes no notes during the assignment conference. She was on the same team with the same assignment yesterday. Mrs. Green has been off duty for three days. She seems more interested in telling Mrs. Evans and Miss Allen about what she did at home for three days than in listening to report. Miss Allen listens to report and assignment conference with half-interest.

Mrs. Crawford makes patient rounds immediately after report and assignment conferences. She spends about one hour making rounds and utilizes the time to meet patient needs and talk with patients. The highlight of patient-care needs on Team 2 is that one patient who was anuric postoperatively is receiving peritoneal dialysis. Mrs. Crawford has assigned this patient to Mrs. Evans, LPN, who has had this experience previously. Mrs. Green, LPN, has never done peritoneal dialysis. Mrs. Green's assignment consists of patient-care needs that are neither new nor particularly challenging. Miss Allen's assignment is relatively light today.

As the day progresses, nursing care is accomplished as planned due to Mrs. Crawford's close supervision. Rather than trying to find team members when something is needed by a patient, Mrs. Crawford meets the need herself. Mrs. Crawford relieves Mrs. Evans, LPN, for lunch since the patient with peritoneal dialysis needs fairly constant care. When relieving her, Mrs. Crawford finds that the peritoneal cycles have been charted incorrectly. She corrects this herself. The patient also complains that she has not yet been bathed and that her skin itches. When Mrs. Evans returns from lunch, Mrs. Crawford says, "Your patient needs skin care; do you remember the special technique we are using for her?"

Team 2 concludes its day with nursing-care objectives met.

An Evaluation Conference

Mrs. Webster has spent most of the day off the unit attending meetings. She returns at 2:00 P.M. and decides that she has enough time to have an annual evaluation conference with one of her staff members. She decides to have one with Mrs. Taber, nurse's aide. Mrs. Webster quickly fills out the rating form and asks Mrs. Taber to come into her office for a few minutes. The evaluation conference goes like this:

MRS. WEBSTER: Mrs. Taber, I have completed your yearly evaluation and thought you would like to read it over. You can sign it at the bottom.

MRS. TABER (*after reading it*): You have me marked below average on "attitude." What's wrong with my attitude?

MRS. WEBSTER: There's nothing wrong with it. It's just that you have a tendency to be sullen at times. Now I know you don't do this often and, as you can see by the other markings, you've really done a good job on 4N. Do you have any questions?"

MRS. TABER: No.

MRS. WEBSTER: Good. Please sign that you've read it. (*Mrs. Taber signs the evaluation and leaves.*)

It is now 3:00 P.M. and time to report to the afternoon shift. Another day shift has come to an end on 4N.

Study Questions

1. Identify the management problems on 4N.
2. What are possible solutions to each problem?
3. Which solution would you choose and why?
4. Considering the personalities of the staff involved, what difficulties would you expect in bringing about changes that might solve the problems?

Eight Hours in the Wardship Hospital Emergency Room

The Wardship Hospital emergency room provides emergency treatment in Wardship, a middle-class residential suburb with a population of 60,000. It serves an average daily census of 60 patients. There are five rooms, each with two beds. This case will describe the people involved and the events occurring on an eight-hour shift from 7:00 A.M. to 3:30 P.M.

Personnel

Miss Plain is the head nurse. Her name serves as a description, as she is quiet, nondynamic, and very mousy in appearance. She has served as head nurse for two months and was previously a staff nurse in another state. Mrs. Clark, RN, has worked in the emergency room for the two years following graduation from nursing school. She is efficient and skilled technically, but is frequently blunt and tactless in communication with staff members and patients. Miss Hambrick, RN, graduated from nursing school one year ago. Her approach to patients is both professional and kind. She uses good judgment in patient care and is interested in learning and helping others to learn quality emergency room nursing care. Two senior student nurses are assigned to the unit for two weeks. Their purpose in the ER is to learn emergency room policy and nursing care through giving patient care under the supervision of their instructor or the staff nurses. The instructor is responsible for five other student nurses scattered throughout the hospital and, therefore, is in the ER at occasional intervals. Both students have studied content about emergency room nursing care, but neither of the two students has been involved in a stressful or true emergency situation. An intern is in the ER 24 hours a day.

The Day's Activities

The day begins with the routine tasks of cleaning the rooms and checking the equipment. At 7:30 A.M. the first patient comes into the ER, with complaints of dizziness and faintness on the way to work.

He is a diabetic who skipped breakfast. After being given some glucose intravenously, he is asked to stay and rest for a few minutes. One of the student nurses was following this patient when the head nurse asked her to take another patient to the x-ray department. The diabetic patient left the ER unnoticed by the staff members before receiving any instructions or teaching.

A 40-year-old woman is admitted next with complaints of epigastric pain. After being seen by the intern, she is asked to wait for further tests and examination. She is apprehensive and uncomfortable. All the nurses peek in the door at intervals to see how she is, but none takes time to try to make her more comfortable. A patient with a broken finger and one with a twisted ankle are also seen before 9:00 A.M. They are treated and discharged.

At 9:00 A.M. the police bring a 70-year-old man who has been involved in a car accident to the ER. He was a driver involved in a head-on collision with another car. The two students and their instructor plan to follow this case. As neurosurgeons, general surgeons, and orthopedic surgeons take their turns with the patient, the students are busy and tense with assisting the doctors. No staff nurse offers to assist. The staff nurses are busy with patients in other rooms, and the head nurse is involved in ordering supplies and doing paperwork. The patient's wife sits alone in a waiting lounge. She is unaware that her husband's condition is critical and growing worse. Each of the specialists treating the patient is concerned only with his specialty. No one is viewing the patient as a total person except for the instructor who is helping the students and growing anxious as she sees the patient's condition worsening. She finds a brief minute to take the patient's valuables to the wife and to explain what is being done for the patient.

At 1:00 P.M. the student nurses and instructor are still with the car accident patient. At this hour he has a cardiac arrest that makes an already chaotic atmosphere catastrophic. The resident at the bedside is hyperactive and nonproductive as he jumps from one thing to another; the student nurses are nervous but functioning fairly well. The instructor is doing what she can to keep a proper perspective on the patient's needs. The head nurse opens the door a crack and makes a hasty exit. Mrs. Clark comes in and is efficient and helpful in getting equipment and drugs assembled. The patient does not respond to treatment and expires. The students, shaken by their first contact with death, assist in postmortem patient care, cleaning the room and equipment, and then welcome a chance to relax and unwind. The instructor, who has not seen the other students for four hours, makes a hasty exit to make rounds. The head nurse begins to complete the death certificate.

At 2:00 P.M. a mother comes to the ER with her son, a one-year-old toddler. He may have swallowed some aspirin, but the mother is not sure. The doctor orders an emetic given and a blood test drawn for salicylate level. When Mrs. Clark attempts to give the child the emetic, the mother says, "Is that really necessary? I'm not sure if he took the aspirin."

Mrs. Clark replies curtly, "The doctor ordered this, but if you want to refuse treatment you can."

The mother says, "But I thought he would want to see the results of the blood test first."

Mrs. Clark replies, "That may take an hour to run, and meanwhile he should have this." The child starts to cry loudly, and the mother is visibly upset. The mother helps the nurse give the child the medicine.

At 3:00 P.M. the nurses, tired from a physically and emotionally traumatic day, complete their day's work in the ER.

Study Questions

1. Identify the management problems in the ER.
2. What are the possible solutions and alternatives to each management problem?
3. How could the solutions best be accomplished?
4. What are the needs for staff development?
5. If you were Miss Hambrick, how would you institute a change in policy?
6. Was this day a learning experience for the student nurses? Could the experience have been handled differently by the instructor and the staff nurses?
7. If you were to help Miss Plain with leadership qualities, where would you begin?
8. How do you think Mrs. Clark would respond to constructive criticism from Miss Plain? Role play an evaluation conference between the two.

Staff Nursing in Transition

Mrs. Healy, the head nurse on a 60-bed, medical-surgical patient-care unit, is an energetic woman who has actively participated in many community events related to her children's school life. She enjoys organizing and likes a flurry of activity, feeling satisfied when deadlines have been met. Mrs. Healy has been the head nurse on this patient-care unit for seven years and has initiated several innovations in nursing-care plans and team conferences. Recently Mrs. Healy has been a member of an advisory committee organized within the nursing department to evaluate the feasibility of initiating the primary care pattern of patient-care assignments.

Of all the committee members, Mrs. Healy is most enthusiastic about the concepts of primary nursing care. She likes the idea of nurses having 24-hour responsibility for patients and supports the involvement of the RN staff in direct care of patients. Because of her enthusiasm, she has volunteered to work with her staff to make the transition from team to primary care along with another head nurse. The second head nurse also has responsibility for a 60-bed, medical-surgical patient-care unit.

The two head nurses have decided to follow a similar methodology in making the transition. Mr. Estrand, the other head nurse, is a calm, soft-spoken person who expresses himself well. In contrast with Mrs. Healy's energetic approach, his seems to be reserved and conservative. In their discussion of methodology for introducing primary nursing, it is clear that the two head nurses prefer different approaches. Mr. Estrand would like to begin by conducting group conferences to engage the staffs of the two units in a study of primary nursing and discuss their expectations of the new pattern of care. Mrs. Healy feels that this approach is a delaying tactic and prefers to draw up guidelines for the new pattern that both head nurses could use.

Mrs. Healy's patient-care unit serves patients with short-term illnesses, many of whom are admitted for gastrointestinal and genitourinary problems. Some of these patients remain in the hospital for two or three days, being admitted for diagnostic procedures. Others have elective short-term surgery. Mr. Estrand's patient-care unit serves patients with cardiovascular and respiratory illnesses. These patients tend to remain in the hospital from six to eight days. The staffing for both patient-care units is similar except that Mrs.

Healy's has more nurse's aides, whereas Mr. Estrand's has more LPNs. Both have about the same number of RNs. Mrs. Healy believes that they should both change their staffing to an all RN staff in order to initiate primary nursing care successfully. Mr. Estrand does not agree. They reach a compromise in that each decides to manage staffing ratios independently and both will use the outline they have prepared to initiate primary care.

For the most part, this outline consists of a new job description for the RN, including a statement of the purpose of primary care, the responsibilities of the RN, and the expected benefits of changing from team to primary nursing care. Mrs. Healy and Mr. Estrand decide to present this outline to their respective staffs independently, and they plan to compare their impressions of the staff responses to determine how they can best support one another during the transition.

Two weeks after presenting the outline to the staff, Mrs. Healy receives resignations from three of the five nurse's aides and three registered nurses. She cannot understand why these people are resigning because her relationships with the staff have always been based on trust and mutual respect. During the two weeks since she initiated the new pattern of primary nursing, the staff has seemed to work effectively. The registered nurses indicate that they like the primary care pattern and state that they prefer being "peers" rather than having to rotate the position of being in charge of a team. Previously there had been three separate teams, each with a team leader, for the 60 patients. An aide and an RN worked with the team leader for each of the teams.

Mr. Estrand does not change staffing to primary care patterns all at once as does Mrs. Healy. Instead, he asks the RNs for volunteers to be primary nurses to "pilot" the transition for the patient-care unit. Only two RNs volunteer, but he thinks this number sufficient and retains the ongoing team nursing staffing pattern for two teams. He reduces the number of staff and patients for the third team to accommodate the primary care "pilot" staffing. Mrs. Healy thinks that his approach is too conservative and secretly wonders whether Mr. Estrand really wants to convert to primary nursing. The two nurses who volunteered to be primary nurses on his unit like their new role and demonstrate their interest by studying primary nursing care literature. Two of the RNs on Mr. Estrand's unit think that primary care will never work, but the remainder of the RNs are watchful.

Mary Smith and Jane Ellis are two of the nurse's aides on Mrs. Healy's patient-care unit who decide that they should resign. They have been checking the positions available that are posted by the personnel department and plan to interview for ward clerk positions. Susan Palmer, another nurse's aide, discusses their plans with them and also decides to resign. She plans to seek employment at a nursing home located near her residence, which is 20 miles from the hospital.

The three RNs who plan to resign from Mrs. Healy's patient-care unit ask to be transferred to other departments in the hospital. One asks for a position in the coronary care unit, so that she can advance her knowledge and experience. The other two are uncertain about what to do. One wants to investigate degree programs in nursing, and the other is thinking about applying for a job as a school nurse.

Mrs. Healy holds conferences with each of the six persons who are transferring or resigning. She challenges the registered nurses with the idea that they are finding primary care difficult and offers to assist them in developing a continuing education program to increase their knowledge. She thinks this approach is appropriate since two of the three RNs tell her that their desire to continue their education is the major reason for resigning. In the conferences with the nurse's aides, Mrs. Healy emphasizes their need for career planning. She hopes to help them find ways to upgrade their education. Although Mrs. Healy is distressed by their abrupt resignations, she is already formulating plans for revising her budget to employ more RNs and fewer nurse's aides. She does not mention her plans to change the budget to anyone.

One registered nurse and two nurse's aides actually terminate their employment at the hospital and are interviewed by the personnel representative in a routine exit interview. The RN tells this representative that she is leaving because the patients are being neglected with the new primary nursing care. She feels that the RN has too many patients in this new method and cannot "be everywhere at once." She says, "In the team method, someone was always free to see a patient or to answer a patient's call." Now each nurse is specifically assigned to certain patients and cannot be available to all the patients. This RN also expresses a feeling of loss about not getting to know all the patients assigned to the team and about not having the help of the aides.

The two nurse's aides who are leaving the hospital tell the personnel representative that they know they should resign because Mrs. Healy is "set on having primary nursing care and doesn't want aides." They express high regard for Mrs. Healy personally, but feel that she has made up her mind and will forge ahead until she accomplishes her goal. They know that the hospital will support Mrs. Healy because primary nursing is the coming thing, and they "may as well accept it" and find something else to do.

Study Questions

1. Compare the approaches used by Mrs. Healy and Mr. Estrand to initiate primary nursing care.
2. Analyze the approaches used by Mrs. Healy and Mr. Estrand in terms of:
   a. The management theories that apply
   b. Reactions of staff members to change
   c. The motivation of each of the head nurses
   d. The possible effects on the patients' care during the transition period
3. Consider that you are applying for a staff nurse position and can select a position with either Mrs. Healy or Mr. Estrand. Which position would you select? Give the rationale for your selection.
4. Evaluate the effects of the six resignations from Mrs. Healy's patient-care area on the following persons:
   a. Mr. Estrand
   b. Mrs. Healy
   c. The staff nurses on both patient-care areas
   d. Other staff nurses working in the hospital
   e. Nurse's aides working on other patient-care units
5. What measures would you suggest that Mr. Estrand and Mrs. Healy take now that would facilitate the transition to primary care from the perspective of the:
   a. Staff nurses
   b. The advisory committee
   c. The Director of Nursing Service
6. Evaluate the potential for the success of the project to initiate primary care nursing staffing patterns in this hospital.

The Case of the Missing Tape Recorder

Walton Community Hospital is located in a community of 5,000 people. The hospital has five patient-care units including obstetrics, a convalescent care unit, and three medical-surgical nursing units. The hospital has an operating room, physical therapy and occupational therapy departments, laboratory and x-ray facilities, and an emergency room. Specialists come to the hospital from a nearby city for consultation and for special services requiring expertise in medical practice. Patients are referred to the larger hospital when their needs require health care services not available at Walton.

Many of the nurses employed by Walton are part-time nurses who fill in when needed for private duty or who work one to three days per week. The full-time staff is made up of a combination of older nurses who have resided in the community all their married lives, and young graduates who plan to work at the hospital for a year or two at most. There are permanent staff nurses for days, evenings, and nights—only occasionally does a staff member have to rotate shifts.

The director of nursing is a relaxed and pleasant individual who likes to become involved in patient-care activities. She knows all the patients, and hospital personnel are accustomed to seeing her in every department of the hospital, as she likes to know how the patients are progressing when they go to surgery, to the lab, to PT or OT, or when they are on the patient-care units. Personnel often comment that her name fits her personality, as she is Mrs. Gladden in her contacts with the patients.

Mrs. Gladden loves gadgets, and new techniques of caring for patients fascinate her. She particularly likes to discuss the "big city" hospital methods with the young graduates who come to Walton to work. Many of the staff members recognize that the director would like to be involved in a "progressive medical center" atmosphere like that of her student experience, but that her home and family ties keep her in Walton.

The five patient-care units are semi-autonomous in methods used to organize staff. The atmosphere of the hospital is informal and there are no supervisors. The title of head nurse has been discontinued and the title, "coordinator," is used instead. Mrs. Gladden had decided that the title "head nurse" was traditional and changed the title to coordinator in order to emphasize the clinical leadership role of the nurse. There are no position descriptions for the coordinators. Two of the five coordinators are having difficulty deciding how to interpret the role of the coordinator because they do not perceive any significant changes in the behaviors of the other three coordinators. One of the two, Mrs. Caller, has been working at Walton for two years. She was formerly a head nurse in a larger hospital where the head nurses were supported and guided by supervisors. She was so accustomed to working in this situation that she finds it difficult to work at Walton as a coordinator, because there are no supervisors. The other coordinator, Mrs. Hill, was appointed to the position after working as a staff nurse at Walton for six months. Since she had never been appointed to a leadership position, she is not sure about what her job entails and does not know if she is "doing the right things" as coordinator.

The other three coordinators have been employees at Walton for fifteen or twenty years and have learned to manage their units in an independent fashion. The coordinator in obstetrics can rightfully boast that she has taken care of every child born in Walton for the last seventeen years. She knows everyone in the community and is often called upon for advice by mothers who are uncertain of what to do during the prenatal and postnatal periods. The doctors on the medical staff depend on her because she is a very capable nurse who knows obstetric theory and practice.

The two other "secure" coordinators are also knowledgeable about patient care and are able to make decisions about patient care. They know the doctors and understand their preferences for care. These three coordinators get along well and often share stories of their units. Other staff members, the newer staff included, enjoy hearing their tales of events of the past which involved some of the doctors currently on the medical staff as well as some of the patients who still come to the hospital.

A new graduate from a nearby school of nursing has recently been employed at the Walton hospital on Mrs. Hill's medical-surgical nursing unit. The graduate, Miss Melton, is alert and enthusiastic about patient care. She feels that Mrs. Hill does not exert enough influence in utilizing new techniques for patient care or for teaching staff. Her opinions were formed during the first weeks of employment when she did not receive an expected orientation to the unit and when most of her questions about what to do were answered with, "We . . . well, what do you think we should do?"

Staff members of the unit include two other RNs, an LPN, and four nurse's aides, one of whom works four days per week, two on the day shift and two on the evening shift. These staff members find Miss Melton refreshing. They enjoy working with her because she has new and "efficient" ways of caring for patients that are sometimes different from the methods usually accepted as the way to do things by the staff. All the staff members have begun to ask questions of Miss Melton instead of the coordinator because she gives quick and definite answers to their questions. All the staff members, that is, except one—the nurse's aide who works two day shifts and two evening shifts per week.

This nurse's aide, Mary Parks, often finds Miss Melton's ways of doing things disconcerting because she never knows what is expected of her. Formerly, she could work days or evenings and know just what to do, but now things are always changing. Mary is considering asking to move to another unit or to work straight evenings, even though she knows that there is no position open on the evening shift.

One of the things that most bothered Mary was the care of a patient who had just discovered he had diabetes. Miss Melton had worked with other staff members to decide how to teach the patient about his diet. They had obtained a scale from the kitchen so that the patient could weigh his food for replacement. Miss Melton thought that if he weighed his food in the hospital, he would be better able to manage his diet at home. Mary had reacted strongly to seeing the scale in the patient's room because it got in her way. She was also upset because the patient asked her to check the accuracy of his weights and she did not know how to read the scale.

Now Mary is upset because the "new" Miss Melton has come up with another bright idea. Because so many personnel work part time, Miss Melton had asked Mrs. Hill if they could get a tape recorder to tape reports. That way she would not have to stop patient care to give reports at 9:00 A.M. and 10:00 A.M. to oncoming staff. Mrs. Hill had been reluctant to ask, but Miss Melton gained her permission to ask Mrs. Gladden for the recorder. As could be expected, Mrs. Gladden was delighted with the idea and immediately procured a tape recorder for the experiment.

Mary conveyed her dislike for Miss Melton and her new ideas to the evening charge nurse, Mrs. Sharp. Her comments were received with thoughtfulness because Mrs. Sharp has great respect for Mary's ability to care for patients. She is precise and pays attention to details in carrying out directions. Mrs. Sharp had misgivings about using the tape recorder anyway, because she felt very strange using a recorder for reports rather than telling the next nurse about the patients in person. She did try the new method for a day or two and then decided that using a tape recorder took too much of her time. She also worried about the tape recorder's being left at the nursing station all evening because the staff was often busy with patient care during the evening, leaving the station unattended. Mrs. Sharp's solution to this problem was to lock the tape recorder in the equipment area. Soon after placing the recorder on a high empty shelf in the locked cabinet, Mrs. Sharp admitted a critically ill patient. In the hurry and stress of the evening she did not give the recorder another thought.

When the night nurse came at 11:00 P.M., Mrs. Sharp gave her a detailed report. The two nurses spent some time with the critically ill patient so that Mrs. Sharp could be sure that the night nurse knew what to do for the patient. The night nurse had been on vacation for the past two weeks and had to be oriented to all the patients very thoroughly. Mrs. Sharp was finally satisfied that the unit was under control and left at 2:00 A.M.

On the following morning Mrs. Hill could not find the tape recorder. The night nurse did not know about the new method and had no idea where the recorder was. After some searching Mrs. Hill determined that the recorder had been stolen. She was concerned because she knew that Mrs. Gladden would be upset about the loss—not only for the tape recorder but also for the apparent failure of the new method for giving reports.

Study Questions

1. How do you think this situation was handled by the following persons?
   a. Mrs. Gladden
   b. Mrs. Hill
   c. Miss Melton
   d. Mrs. Sharp
   e. Mary Parks
   f. The other members of the nursing staff
2. Identify the problems which are inherent in this case in reference to:
   a. The hospital organization
   b. The nursing-department
   c. The organization of the patient-care unit
   d. Relationships among staff members
   e. Needs of the staff for staff development
3. How would you have handled yourself in this situation had you been Miss Melton?
4. Outline the solutions for the problems identified. Be specific in determining a course of action for all the staff who play prominent roles in this situation.

Index

Index